Alternatives
for
Women with Endometriosis

Alternatives

for

Women with Endometriosis

A Guide by Women for Women

Ruth Carol, editor

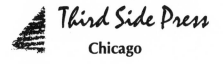

Third Side Press
Chicago

The ideas and suggestions contained in this book are not intended as a substitute for consulting with a medical physician and/or holistic practitioner.

Library of Congress Cataloging-in-Publication Data
Alternatives for women with endometriosis : a guide by women for women
  / Ruth Carol, editor.
     p. cm.
   Includes bibliographical references and index.
   ISBN 1-879427-15-X (cloth) . — ISBN 1-879427-12-5 (pbk.).
   1. Endometriosis—Alternative treatment.   2. Endometriosis—
Popular works.   I. Carol, Ruth, 1964-
RG483.E53A45   1994
618.1—dc20   94-10122
                                                         CIP

Third Side Press
2250 W. Farragut
Chicago, IL 60625-1802

First edition, August 1994
10 9 8 7 6 5 4 3 2

To my mother and grandmother,
who have nurtured me throughout my life
and continue to do so.

To my husband, Glenn,
who has supported me in all of my endeavors.

To my daughter, Ashley,
for showing me there are such things as miracles.

Contents

Introduction

You've been here. Your legs are high in the stirrups on the table in the gynecologist's office. You're trying to peer over the white *gown* that feels more like cheap toilet paper, to look at the doctor while he or she—usually he—tells you everything appears normal. And why are you having so much pain during your periods, and perhaps between your periods?

"Some women have painful periods," the doctor concludes, writing out a prescription for more painkillers. Or maybe this time, you're told that the pain is stress-related. The *prescription*: relax, cut back on your busy schedule, or see *someone* about your problems. Before you can ask another question, the doctor is out the door.

Eventually you learn that your pain has a name—*endometriosis*. Endometriosis is a disease in which the tissue that normally lines the inside of the uterus travels outside of it. This tissue adheres to the various abdominal organs, usually the ovaries, the fallopian tubes, and the uterosacral ligaments. The bowel and bladder are often involved as well. The endometrial tissue takes the form of implants, lesions, cysts, and nodules. Like the endometrium that remains on the inside of the uterus, the displaced tissue responds to your hormonal cycles and breaks down and bleeds

9

each month. But this blood is trapped inside the pelvic cavity. Over time, these implants can form scar tissue and adhesions that cause pelvic pain, menstrual cramping, painful intercourse, infertility, and gastrointestinal problems, to name a few.

To date, there is no known cause or cure for endometriosis. The mainstream medical treatments for it—drugs and surgery—are often costly and temporary.

For years, women with endometriosis have been treated with Danocrine (danazol), which puts the body in a state of pseudo-menopause. Although the drug is generally successful in treating endometriosis, this synthetic testosterone derivative has a host of masculinating side effects, including decreased breast size, facial hair growth, and deepening of the voice. Other common side effects include hot flashes, night sweats, weight gain, edema, headaches, acne, oily skin, vaginal dryness, mood swings, and depression. The majority of women taking danazol experience some of these side effects, and the androgenic ones may not reverse once the drug is discontinued. Danazol is typically prescribed for three to nine months and can cost more than $200 a month, depending on the dosage. Moreover, the endometriosis symptoms can recur shortly after treatment is discontinued. Clinical studies have shown that half of patients have recurring symptoms within one year of being off danazol.

More recently, women with endometriosis have been successfully treated with gonadotrophin-releasing hormone (GnRH) analogs, which also lower the hormones to post-menopausal levels. The GnRH analogs currently come in two forms: Lupron (leuprolide acetate; a monthly injection) and Synarel (nafarelin acetate; a nasal spray). Like danazol, GnRH analogs have no effect on adhesions or scar tissue, but unlike danazol, GnRH analogs do not have masculinating side effects. However, they do produce menopausal side effects, namely hot flashes, vaginitis, and decreased libido. Then there is the other side effect—bone density loss—some of which may not be reversible after treatment with the drug has stopped. Treatment is typically six months, and the cost is in the $300-a-month range. The endometriosis symptoms sometimes recur within months after treatment is discontinued.

Some women are unable to tolerate the side effects of these drugs and therefore cannot take them. Others may not be good candidates for the drugs. For example, women who suffer from kidney or liver dysfunction, smoke, or have migraines or a family history of osteoporosis should not be taking the drugs. Many women who do not have medical insurance or who are not covered because their endometriosis is considered a preexisting condition cannot afford the drugs. Then there are those who are trying to conceive. Taking a drug that suppresses the hormones and menstrual cycle obviously and significantly decreases the possibility of conception.

For women who *can* tolerate them, the drugs offer only temporary relief from the symptoms because they are prescribed for just three, six, or nine months at a time. The GnRH analogues can be prescribed for up to six months, initially, and danazol can be initially prescribed for up to nine months. Although danazol can be prescribed for an additional nine-month therapy, the GnRH analogs are not recommended for a second round of treatment because safety data beyond six months are unavailable. (It is also possible to use one drug for a while and then the other, but even with a strategy like that you run out of drug therapy in about two years.)

With drugs ruled out, women with endometriosis may turn to the other conventional medical treatment for endometriosis—surgery. Currently, the only way to definitively diagnose endometriosis is through a laparoscopy, a surgical procedure performed under anesthesia, usually on an outpatient basis. During a laparoscopy, implants and endometriomas can be lasered, excised, cauterized, or vaporized to bring about pain relief successfully. However, disease can be either microscopic or atypical in appearance and therefore missed, and new growths can occur. Furthermore, adhesions can begin reforming as soon as the incisions are stitched up. Some women resort to undergoing surgery every couple of years to maintain tolerable pain levels. Laser laparoscopy is an increasingly popular choice because it is precise (when in the hands of a well-trained and skilled physician) and reduces bleeding and formation of postoperative scar tissue and adhesions. This type of surgery typically costs approximately $2,500 or more, depending on the extent of the disease.

Between the costs and the risks inherent in the mainstream medical treatments for endometriosis, many women have reason to seek alternative therapies. Among the type of therapies for endometriosis discussed in this book are nutrition, vitamin supplementation, herbal remedies, Traditional Chinese Medicine, homeopathy, naturopathy, chiropractic, candida treatment, clinical ecology, exercise, yoga, massage therapy, and visualization.

Mainstream Skepticism

The mainstream medical profession is skeptical, to say the least, of alternative therapies. Typical comments from physicians about these therapies include "There's no conclusive evidence that it works" and "Well, as long as it doesn't hurt you."

To some degree, the medical profession cannot help its skepticism. After all, alternative therapies have not undergone double-blind, randomized clinical trials, which are standard in allopathic medical research. But if the mainstream physicians knew more about holistic medicine, they would understand that these therapies do not lend themselves to clinical trials. Because holistic practitioners treat the patient as a whole—incorporating physical symptoms with emotional and spiritual factors—they offer very individualized treatments, and no two people are treated the same. Consequently, holistic practitioners would not think of dividing a group of women with endometriosis and providing the *same* treatment to half and a placebo to the other half. More likely they would provide unique treatments with overlapping aspects to all. Besides, what kind of placebo do you substitute for an acupuncture needle? Furthermore, why would the pharmaceutical industry fund clinical trials that may prove the existence of a less costly, less toxic alternative to the drugs currently on the market?

As more scientific studies suggest reasons alternative therapies work, such as acupuncture needles stimulate the release of endorphins (the body's natural painkillers), the mainstream medical profession's skepticism may slowly give way to more acceptance of unconventional therapies.

To that end, the Office for the Study of Alternative Medicine was established by the National Institutes of Health in 1992. With a $3.5 million budget in 1994, the office is charged with developing strategies to scientifically evaluate alternative therapies. Among those being investigated are visualization for asthma

patients, acupuncture for hyperactive children, and
biofeedback for chronic back pain.

Another sign of this growing acceptance is that some
medical schools have begun offering courses on
alternative medicine. Among them are Harvard
Medical School, University of California at San
Francisco, University of Maryland, University of
Virginia, University of Arizona, University of
Louisville, Georgetown University, and the University
of Massachusetts in Worcester. In fact, the Stress
Reduction Clinic at the University of Massachusetts in
Worcester and the Mind/Body Medical Institute at
Deaconess Hospital in Boston offer classes on
meditation and yoga to patients for ailments from
infertility and gastrointestinal disorders to AIDS and
cancer. Although the mainstream medical hardliners
will probably always be critical of the effectiveness of
alternative therapies, one can hope that allopathic
physicians and holistic practitioners can at least
develop a mutual respect in the future.

Even if most allopathic physicians show little
interest in alternative therapies, that is not stopping
their patients from doing so. According to a study
published in the January 28, 1993, issue of *The New
England Journal of Medicine* one in three Americans
(out of 1,539 interviewed) had used an unconventional
therapy in the previous year. Moreover, one third of
the respondents routinely saw alternative practitioners
for such treatments, making an average of 19 visits
annually, with an average charge of $27.60 per visit.

According to the study, educated, upper-income
white Americans, ranging in age from 25 to 49, are the
most frequent users of alternative therapies. The
majority of respondents used alternative therapies
(such as relaxation techniques, chiropractic, and
massage therapy) for chronic conditions, including

back problems, anxiety, and headaches. Other
unconventional therapies cited include imagery,
spiritual healing, lifestyle diets, herbal medicine,
megavitamin therapy, and homeopathy. Other
conditions for which the respondents sought treatment
include cancer, allergies, digestive problems, arthritis,
and insomnia. Of those who used these therapies for
serious medical ailments, the vast majority also
consulted a medical doctor for the same condition.
Not surprisingly, the majority of respondents who used
unconventional therapies did so without telling their
medical physicians.

When the study figures are extrapolated to the U.S.
population as a whole, they suggest that Americans
made an estimated 425 million visits to holistic
practitioners, spending nearly $14 billion in 1990, the
bulk of which was paid out of pocket. This compared
with 388 million visits that were made to all primary
care physicians nationwide and almost $13 billion
spent out of pocket for all hospitalizations in the
country that same year. The authors of the study
conclude that the use of unconventional therapies in
the United States is much greater than previously
reported.

A 1991 survey taken for *Time* magazine/CNN had
similar results. More than 30 percent of the 500
people polled had sought some form of alternative
therapy in the previous year. Of those who used
alternative therapies, 84 percent would return to the
holistic practitioner. More than 60 percent of those
questioned who did not seek alternative treatments
would do so, if mainstream medicine failed them.

Using This Book

The aim of this book is not to point out where
allopathic medicine has failed, but rather where
holistic medicine has triumphed. The purpose of the
book is to share alternative therapies that have worked
for others in the hope that they may work for you. The
women who have so graciously agreed to share their
experiences not only discuss the specific alternative
therapies they have used to treat (and some say cure)
their endometriosis, but relate their journey in finding
these therapies. Although when faced with more of the
same conventional treatments these women chose to
seek an alternate way of treating their disease, most
still maintain a relationship with both a medical
physician and holistic practitioner(s). That way, they
can get the best of both treatment worlds.

Although they used different and varying alternative
therapies, these women have many things in common.
Foremost, they are living a pain-free existence, or close
to it, despite endometriosis being labeled a chronic
disease. They have worked and continue to work hard
at maintaining this status. These women typically
started by using one alternative therapy and ended up
incorporating a few therapies by the time they settled
on a regimen. Having taken an active role in their
health maintenance, they have formed partnerships
with their holistic practitioners. Finally, these women
have taken control of their own well-being, probably
the most gratifying outcome of all.

It is hoped that the book will be used as an
educational tool because an educated patient is a wise
one who can make good choices about her health care.
I encourage you to read these firsthand experiences
and decide for yourself which therapies will fit into
your lifestyle and work best for you. Naturally, this

book does not substitute for consultation with a doctor or holistic health care provider.

Once you have decided that alternative medicine is an essential key to your good health, the next step is to find a holistic practitioner in your area. Although word-of-mouth can be a good way to find a practitioner, you should make sure this practitioner is licensed by the appropriate board(s). Only a handful of states have medical boards for holistic practitioners, such as homeopaths and naturopaths. However, there are several national certification boards, including the American Academy of Medical Acupuncture, the National Commission for the Certification of Acupuncturists, the National Center for Homeopathy, the American Chiropractic Association, the American Holistic Medical Association, and the American Association of Naturopathic Physicians.

Good luck on your journey toward good health.

Part 1

Alternative Therapies: Theory in Brief

Part 1 offers an overview of the alternative therapies described by the women who share their experiences in Part 2. These brief descriptions discuss the benefits such therapies have been known to have in treating women with endometriosis. These synopses, along with the women's stories, and the bibliographies, which list books for further reading, are pieces to the puzzle of health. I hope that they will help you find the therapy that works best for you.

Chapter 1

Nutrition

Many women with endometriosis report that they
have experienced significant pain relief from changes
in their diet. These include making new food choices as
well as taking vitamins, minerals, and other
supplements. The idea is to make food and supplement
choices that will lower estrogen levels and boost the
immune system.

In general, diet recommendations for women with
endometriosis are aimed at reducing and then
maintaining normal estrogen levels. The liver is largely
responsible for converting estradiol, an active form of
estrogen, into estriol, a safer form of the hormone. In
order to function properly, the liver needs a rich supply
of B vitamins. But many foods deplete the body of B
vitamins. These include refined sugars, processed
foods, saturated (animal) fats, caffeine, salt, and
alcohol. When the liver is stressed, its ability to break
down estrogen is impaired.

Processed foods, refined sugar, salt, animal fats,
alcohol, caffeine, meat, and dairy products should be
eliminated or substantially reduced from the diet. If a
woman with endometriosis must eat meat or poultry,
buying organic meat made from animals that have not
been exposed to hormones, antibiotics, and pesticides
is often suggested. In addition to depleting the body of

B vitamins, all of these promote the production of the *bad* prostaglandins. Prostaglandins are hormone-like substances that cause the contraction of smooth muscles, including the uterus. Uterine contractions are responsible for some of the pain associated with endometriosis. But there are also *good* prostaglandins that studies have shown stop the restriction of blood vessels, breast inflammation, and water retention as well as prevent blood clots. They counteract the effects of the bad prostaglandins. Essential fatty acids, which encourage the production of good prostaglandins, must be provided in the diet because our bodies do not produce them.

Women with endometriosis are encouraged to increase their intake of complex carbohydrates and high-fiber foods, such as whole grains, vegetables, fruits, fish, seeds, and nuts. These foods are excellent sources of B vitamins, vitamins C and E, magnesium, calcium, and potassium, all of which help reduce menstrual cramps. However, whole wheat and citrus fruits can be problematic because of their tendency to be allergens and to raise estrogen levels. Fish, seeds and nuts are also high in essential fatty acids.

Vitamins

Women with endometriosis have benefited from taking B-complex vitamins because of the ability of these vitamins to lower excessive levels of estrogen. The B-complex vitamins include B-1, B-2, B-3, B-6, pantothenic acid, biotin, folic acid, choline, inositol, and para-aminobenzoic acid (PABA). Studies have shown that B-6 in particular reduces menstrual pain and cramps, and helps the body make the *good* prostaglandins. In addition to playing a significant role in the liver function and synthesis of estrogen, the

B-complex vitamins increase energy because they break down carbohydrates. The B-complex vitamins also strengthen the immune system, reduce stress, combat fatigue, and help prevent fluid retention. Both vitamins A and C are known to reduce heavy menstrual bleeding and to boost the immune system. They help promote healing and provide greater resistance to disease. Vitamin A in the form of beta-carotene is often suggested because it is from vegetables, not animals, and therefore not toxic in large amounts. Vitamin C may also help minimize scarring and inflamation. Vitamin E keeps scar tissue soft and flexible and may even minimize scar tissue and adhesions. It breaks down estrogen when there is too much and emulsifies the blood. All vitamins work in conjunction with minerals. The minerals most often mentioned in relation to reducing menstrual cramps are magnesium, calcium, potassium, selenium, and zinc. Magnesium helps by increasing calcium absorption and producing the good prostaglandins. Calcium relieves cramps by keeping the muscles toned, while potassium helps by regulating muscle contraction. Selenium and zinc strengthen the immune system. Selenium, an anti-oxidant, also emulsifies the blood.

Lactobicillus acidophilus, a friendly source of intestinal bacteria, helps maintain normal levels of intestinal flora. An imbalance of intestinal flora can contribute to candida and diarrhea. (See chapter 4 for more information about candida.) Antibiotics, which are typically prescribed for yeast infections, destroy this beneficial intestinal flora. Lactobicillus acidophilus can help digestive problems and restore the acid-base balance in a reproductive system that has been altered by hormonal changes.

When choosing a vitamin regimen, it is important to understand that vitamins interrelate. Taking the appropriate amount of each vitamin in combination with other vitamins is critical. In addition to consulting a nutritionist, you may want to read some books that detail vitamin use, including their individual benefits, best natural sources, and recommended dosages. Several are listed in the Selected Bibliography at the back of this book.

Evening Primrose Oil

Evening primrose oil (EPO) has been proven to relieve pain associated with endometriosis and premenstrual syndrome (PMS), which many women with endometriosis also suffer from. EPO is a natural source of gamma-linoleic acid (GLA), an essential fatty acid that encourages the production of the good prostaglandins, and it has the added benefit of strengthening the immune system.

Excess amounts of prostaglandins are believed to contribute to menstrual difficulties, including cramping, vomiting, headaches, and blood clots, as well as diarrhea and dizziness. Some studies have shown that women with endometriosis produce more prostaglandins than women who do not have the disease (Badawy, 1982). Other studies have shown that women who have PMS produce less GLA than women who do not have this syndrome. The former women also produce excess amounts of the chemicals that the body uses to produce the bad prostaglandins.

The fact that many women get pain relief from taking nonsteroidal anti-inflammatory agents is another indication that prostaglandins play a key role in endometriosis pain. These agents—mefanamic acid, naproxen, ibuprofen, and naproxen sodium, to name a few—work by inhibiting the production of bad prostaglandins and reducing inflammation.

Dietary factors that may impede one's ability to produce GLA include animal fat, dairy products, and caffeine. A diet rich in animal fats contributes to the production of the bad prostaglandins, as does caffeine.

To maximize the benefit of EPO, magnesium, B6, zinc, and vitamin C should be increased, because these help produce GLA. Essential fatty acids can also be found in borage, black currant, and fish oils.

Chapter 2

Herbalism

Herbalism is the oldest natural healing method. Long before allopathic drugs were around, herbal medicines were being made from flowers, roots, leaves, stems, seeds, and bark. In fact, ingredients for many allopathic drugs were derived from herbs. Once these properties could be synthetically reproduced, allopathic medicines replaced herbs. However, herbalists maintain that herbs are superior to allopathic drugs because herbs neither usually cause side effects nor are they addictive. In addition, the entire plant is used in herbal remedies for maximum therapeutic effect. Conventional drugs are typically made of only the active ingredient of a particular plant, discounting the other components as necessary for healing.

Herbal remedies can be taken in the form of a tea, tablet, tincture, infusion, ointment, lotion, or suppository. How the remedy will be prepared and administered depends largely on the type of herb(s) being used and the condition to be treated. Typically, several herbs (anywhere from five to fifteen) are combined for remedies to provide maximum benefit.

Because the remedies are prepared for each individual, no two women with endometriosis would receive exactly the same remedy, even if they have the same symptoms. Furthermore, because the remedies are made based on what the individual needs at a particular point in time, it is unlikely that the same remedy would be repeated. In addition to formulating remedies, an herbalist or a naturopath or homeopath with herbal training also offers dietary advice and even addresses lifestyle changes in an attempt to help restore balance in the whole person.

Herbal remedies have been known to decrease menstrual pain. Remedies for women with endometriosis should focus on reducing estrogen levels, regulating hormonal production, controlling heavy flow, and calming pain. Herbs providing relief for endometriosis include vitex berries, motherwort, black or blue cohosh, red raspberry, red clover, and cayenne. Goldenseal and shepherd's purse help control heavy menstrual bleeding. White willow and meadowsweet can reduce pain and inflammation. Wild yam can help alleviate low abdominal pain. Chamomile flowers, balm, melilot, and rosemary may relieve pain right before or during menses.

Bach Flower Remedies

Bach flower remedies, one particular type of herbal remedies, are prepared from flowering plants and trees. Dr. Edward Bach, a homeopath, believed that negative states of mind make the body vulnerable to disease. He developed 38 remedies that are used to treat the negative emotions responsible for a particular physical disorder. The remedies cover what Bach felt were all the negative states of mind: fear, uncertainty, lack of interest in the present, despondency and despair, overconcern for the welfare of others, loneliness, and oversensitivity. Some Bach flower remedies that may be appropriate for women with endometriosis include Gorse, for feelings of hopelessness and futility; Olive, for mental and physical exhaustion, which may present after an illness or personal ordeal; and Sweet Chestnut, for those who feel they have reached their limits of endurance. Bach flower remedies are often used in conjunction with emotional counseling to assist in the natural healing process.

Chapter 3

Traditional Chinese Medicine

Traditional Chinese Medicine (TCM) has been used to treat menstrual problems, including dysmenorrhea and infertility, for more than 5000 years. TCM strives to restore and maintain a balance of chi (pronounced chee and translated to mean energy or life force) in the body. It does so by using acupuncture and herbs.

According to TCM, chi runs through our bodies along pathways called meridians. When chi flows undisturbed along these meridians, a person is healthy. But when chi becomes weakened or impeded by a blockage or stagnation, illness or pain sets in.

Acupuncture

Acupuncture needles are used to stimulate energy points along the meridians to rid them of the imbalance or blockage and to get chi flowing freely once again. These hair-thin steel needles, which should be disposable, are inserted about 1/4 inch into the skin. Typically eight to twelve needles are inserted and left in place anywhere from 20 to 45 minutes. Sometimes the acupuncturist may twist the needles a little to stimulate a point. Although the procedure is relatively painless, a slight sensation may be felt when the needle is inserted or rotated.

An acupuncturist will use observation, listening, questioning, and pulse taking to diagnose endometriosis. Specifically, the acupuncturist will observe the tongue, analyzing its color, form, degree of moisture, coating, and motility. It is thought that the tongue reveals the nature of a disease. Pulse taking can take a while as there are nearly 30 pulses recognized in TCM.

Although each case is unique, with varying symptoms and diagnoses, endometriosis is generally regarded in TCM as stagnated chi and blood. The treatment goal is to unblock the meridians and release the blockage. The prescribed herbs aim is to help regulate the hormones.

Studies have shown that acupuncture works to significantly reduce menstrual pain, including cramps, nausea, headache, backache, breast tenderness, and fluid retention. In addition, women have reduced their use of nonsteroidal anti-inflammatory agents by using acupuncture (Helms, 1987).

Chinese Herbs

Chinese herbs are used in conjunction with acupuncture to detoxify and strengthen the body. Traditional Chinese herbs resemble pieces of root or bark that must be boiled in a tea. However, many Chinese herbs have been patented and made into pill form. These pills are typically much larger than the pills purchased at the pharmacy, and usually several must be taken at one time. Dong quai is a Chinese herb commonly used to treat menstrual disorders, including cramps.

Several studies from China have shown that the majority of women with endometriosis who took Chinese herbs received significant pain relief. Pelvic pain and pain experienced during intercourse were also relieved (Dharmananda, 1993). In a U.S. study, many women reported that they experienced significant pain relief and that their cycles became more regular when they were taking Chinese herbs (Shattuck, 1993).

Chapter 4

Homeopathy, Naturopathy, Chiropractic

Homeopathy, naturopathy, and chiropractic are three
types of holistic therapies. As such, all three recognize
the importance of physical, emotional, and spiritual
factors in the assessment of health. Consequently, these
therapies offer very individualized treatments for
women with endometriosis. Although the specific
philosophies behind them vary, all three aim to identify
and treat the cause of the illness, rather than simply
suppress the symptoms.

Homeopathy

Homeopathy is based on the Law of Similars, that is,
like cures like. A homeopathic remedy is a substance
that when given in a large amount produces symptoms
in a healthy person; it is given in a minute amount to
treat a sick person suffering from those symptoms. A
homeopathic remedy triggers the body's ability to fight
whatever is causing the symptoms. In that sense,
homeopathy is similar to vaccines, which are minute
amounts of killed virus that stimulate the body's
immune system to prepare to fight off a disease.
Homeopathic remedies, which are made from animal,

mineral, or vegetable substances, come in dilutions or pellets and are based on each individual's symptoms. Homeopaths do not believe in surgery or prescription drugs and are trained in herbalism and nutrition. Homeopathic remedies that may be recommended for endometriosis—depending on an individual's symptoms, emotions, and spirits—include china, nux vomica, graphites, phosophorus, sepia, chamomila, calcarea carbonica, urtica urens, caulophyllum, cocculus, gelsmium, cimicifuga, belladonna, or colocynthis.

Naturopathy

Naturopathy maintains that all diseases are due to the same cause: an accumulation of toxins in the body as a result of an unhealthy lifestyle. Imbalances in the body's structure and emotional stresses can contribute to the buildup of toxins. The goal of naturopathic treatment is twofold: to rid the body of toxins and to rebuild the immune system for good health. To detoxify the body and restore wellness, naturopaths use a variety of natural modalities, including fasting, nutritional and herbal supplements, spinal manipulation, relaxation techniques, hydrotherapy, meditation, and exercise programs.

After the initial fast is over, a naturopath may prescribe a diet high in raw foods, unrefined carbohydrates, and limited protein. Bee pollen, a whole food remedy, may be prescribed for women with endometriosis; it is known to help menstrual problems, to aid in digestion and circulation, and to boost the immune system. Bee pollen works by balancing the hormones and regulating the menstrual cycle. It contains B-complex vitamins, vitamins C and E, and essential fatty acids. Another naturopathic remedy is garlic, which is particularly helpful for healing systemic *Candida albicans*, vaginal yeast infections, and recurrent bladder infections. Castor oil used in heated packs nightly can relieve abdominal cramps. Spinal misalignments can be fixed using either massage techniques, or osteopathic or chiropractic treatments.

Chiropractic

Chiropractic maintains that misalignment of the spinal column causes pressure on the nerves, interfering with the body's ability to function properly and that this misalignment results in disease. Chiropractors use spinal manipulation to realign the spine and thus improve nerve function. Chiropractors who use only adjustments are known as *straights*. Those who also incorporate physical therapy, nutritional recommendations, and counseling are called *mixers*. Kinesiology is a form of chiropractic that uses muscle testing to diagnose the body's weaknesses and deficiencies. Some chiropractors also practice homeopathy and herbalism.

Although chiropractors tend to be consulted for back and neck pain, a poorly aligned spinal column can trigger referred pain in the legs, arms, or internal organs, such as the uterus or intestines. In fact, mechanical disorders of the lumbar spine have been shown to cause pelvic pain. Women with endometriosis may benefit from chiropractic treatment that focuses on restoring normal mobility in the pelvis and reducing soft-tissue strain.

Chapter 5

Immune System-Related Treatments

Although the cause of endometriosis is unknown, one theory about its origin that is gaining acceptance is that it is an immune system dysfunction. This theory suggests that women with endometriosis have an impaired immune system that allows endometrial tissue to grow outside the uterus, wrecking havoc on nearby pelvic organs. In a healthy woman, the immune system would produce cells to prevent the endometrial implants from invading the pelvis. Whether endometriosis is a disease itself or merely a symptom of a more encompassing immunological disorder is yet undetermined. What is certain is that studies suggesting that endometriosis is associated with immune system dysfunction continue to emerge (Rier, 1992).

Moving beyond the pelvis, many women with endometriosis report having immune-system-related illnesses, including chronic yeast infections and allergy-related diseases. The latter include asthma, eczema, allergies, and food intolerances. In addition, many women with endometriosis are relating that they have sensitivities to chemical fumes, such as household cleaners, laundry soaps, perfumes, and cigarette smoke. Most recently, endometriosis has also been linked to environmental pollutants, such as herbicides and industrial wastes. This may mean that endometriosis can be a symptom of environmental illness, or it may mean that women with endometriosis are particularly vulnerable to environmental illness.

Candida

The fact that many women with endometriosis have responded well to an anti-candida program raises a question about a link between endometriosis and yeast. *Candida albicans*, a species of yeast, inhabits all humans. The immune system is charged with keeping it in check. But if the immune system is impaired or malfunctioning, candida can run amok throughout the body, particularly in the intestines, vagina, and mouth. Factors contributing to an overgrowth of yeast include birth control pills (which are often prescribed for women with endometriosis), antibiotics (which are typically prescribed for yeast infections), and pregnancy. As the yeast colonies multiply, they release toxins throughout the body that weaken the immune system.

As part of a typical anti-candida program, nystatin and ketaconazole are two drugs prescribed to reduce yeast colonies. Vitamin supplements and diet changes also focus on ridding the body of excess candida. Studies have shown that women with yeast-related illnesses tend to be deficient in vitamins A, B-3 and B-6, magnesium and zinc, as well as essential fatty acids (such as those found in evening primrose oil).

Eating yogurt, which contains acidophilus, or taking lactobacillus acidophilus tablets, can help. Acidophilus maintains normal amounts of intestinal flora, one of which is yeast. A low-carbohydrate diet kills off the yeast because it cannot thrive on only proteins and fats. It does thrive on overprocessed foods and all forms of sugar, so those should be eliminated. In addition, bread, cheese, vinegar, alcohol, coffee, tea, and smoked meats should be avoided or at least limited. Do these supplements and diet recommendations ring a bell? They should.

Clinical Ecology

A growing number of women with endometriosis report sensitivities to environmental chemicals, which fall under the area of clinical ecology. Practitioners of clinical ecology believe that disease may be caused by sensitivities to foods or chemicals, or both, in the environment. They believe that these sensitivities are responsible for general symptoms, ranging from aches and pains, headaches, fatigue, stuffed sinuses, and irritability to more serious symptoms, such as yeast infections, migraines, and bladder problems—symptoms not typically associated with allergies. Diagnosing these sensitivities is a lengthy process and may involve scratch testing, blood tests, hair analysis, or ingesting or inhaling small amounts of the suspected food(s) or chemical(s) to see whether a problem arises. Another diagnostic tool is the allergy elimination diet, which involves eliminating suspected foods from the diet and reintroducing them one at a time to see if a problem recurs. Many times, the culinary culprit is a familiar food that has been eaten for a prolonged period of time. Foods can either be eliminated from or rotated in the diet. The patient must either avoid the substances identified as problematic or be treated to be less sensitive to them.

Chapter 6

Body Work

Exercise, yoga, and massage therapy can help women
with endometriosis by relieving pain, improving
circulation, and reducing stress. Feldenkrais
neuro-muscular re-education and *t'ai chi ch'uan* are
additional types of body movement taught by
specialized practitioners and used by some women
with endometriosis to improve their physical
well-being.

Exercise

Exercise is known to release endorphins, which are the
body's natural painkillers. Exercise can also prevent
pain by increasing circulation. In fact, poor circulation
in the pelvis could contribute to endometriosis. In
addition, exercise reduces stress and provides more
energy. Exercises that emphasize deep, slow abdominal
breathing have been known to relieve menstrual
cramps by increasing pelvic circulation and reducing
uterine swelling. In addition, exercises designed to
stretch the spine relieve backache. For all of these
reasons, women with endometriosis have experienced
pain relief by establishing an exercise regimen.

Exercises that emphasize stretching and increased
flexibility, rather than going for the burn, are more

beneficial for women with endometriosis for two reasons. One, adhesions can make large, quick movements difficult and uncomfortable. Two, stretching types of exercise can strengthen the back and abdominal muscles. Walking, biking, and swimming are good examples of exercises from which women with endometriosis may gain particular benefit.

Yoga

Although yoga is more than just an exercise, it does have benefits similar to those of exercise. Yoga increases flexibility and circulation, while it strengthens the back and tones the muscles. Like exercise, yoga promotes relaxation and overall well-being. This nonaerobic form of exercise focuses on deep, rhythmic breathing and postures that are held for a specified length of time.

Different postures may be helpful at different times of the menstrual cycle. For example, the corpse pose may reduce premenstrual tension if done in the early stages of the cycle, whereas the pelvic tilt may relieve lower back pain during menses. Other postures that may relieve menstrual pain associated with endometriosis include the half shoulder stand, the locust, the bow, the cobra, the plow, the cat, and the posterior stretch, as well as the child's pose and the wide-angle pose.

Massage Therapy

Massage therapy involves using specific forms of touch to manipulate the body's muscles and soft tissues for healing purposes. It is used to relieve pain, stimulate circulation, and increase range of motion and flexibility of joints. On an emotional level, massage

can reduce anxiety and relieve stress. Forms of massage therapy that can relieve pain for women with endometriosis include acupressure, scar tissue integration therapy, and therapeutic touch.
Acupressure, also known as *shiatsu* in Japanese, is based on the principles of acupuncture. Only instead of needles, the practitioner uses the fingers to stimulate energy points along the meridians to promote healing. A practitioner may hold, rub, or press an area of discomfort, in addition to applying deep finger pressure.
Scar tissue integration therapy works to soften scar tissue, resulting in a greater range of motion. This can be particularly helpful for women with endometriosis, many of whom develop bands of scar tissue, or *adhesions*, that have been known to bind together pelvic organs. Using scar tissue therapy, a therapist would first work to soften tissue tightness. Over time, the therapist would apply more pressure to further soften and stretch the tissue. Once the therapist determines which bands are causing the restricting movement or pain, he or she can work to break the bands, freeing the pelvic organs.
Therapeutic touch is a form of massage that does not involve actual touching. The practitioner holds his or her hands over the patient's body to scan for blockages in its energy fields. The theory behind it is that the body's tissue retains memories. Therapeutic touch can cause those memories to resurface, allowing a patient to deal with them on an emotional basis.

Chapter 7
Visualization

Relaxation techniques, such as visualization and
guided imagery, have been helpful to women with
endometriosis in controlling their pain. Using
visualization techniques, they can mentally remove the
source of pain, resulting in a healing effect on the body.
Visualization involves the use of mental imagery for
a therapeutic purpose. To effectively use visualization,
one must set a goal, create a clear mental picture, focus
on it often, and think about it in positive terms. These
visualization sessions should last anywhere from
fifteen to thirty minutes and should be done at least
three times a day. Women can visualize getting the
endometriosis out of their body, seeing the adhesions
dissolve and atrophy, or imagine white blood cells
attacking the endometriomas. The more detailed the
mental picture, the better. The final image can be a
clear, healthy, pink pelvic cavity, with free flowing
fallopian tubes and spotless ovaries.

Imagery can also be used to set a serene scene in
which the user is free of any aches. This type of
imagery can help one escape the physical pain at least
temporarily.

Positive, strong statements, known as *affirmations*,
reinforce the positive pictures created using
visualization and imagery. Affirmations replace the

negative thoughts that may be lurking in the
unconscious mind, perhaps negatively influencing a
woman's ability to heal herself. Affirmations should be
practiced daily and can be spoken aloud, said silently,
or written down. Affirmations should be phrased in
the present tense, short, simple, and specific to each
individual. Women with endometriosis may want to
use affirmations that focus on their ability to heal
themselves, such as "Every day my pelvis is stronger
and better" or focus on their sexual identity, such as "I
love myself and my body" or "I love being a woman."

Part 2

Our Experience

Part 2 provides firsthand experiences of women with endometriosis who have used alternative therapies to treat their disease. First these women relate the circumstances that led to seeking an alternative therapy, and then they discuss the alternative therapies that they have used to treat (and some say cure) their endometriosis.

Alternative Therapy for Endometriosis

Jo-Ann Allan *21*
Tacoma, Washington
Diagnosed with endometriosis in 1988

Numerous hormone therapies, including (nafarelin acetate) and Lupron (leuprolide acetate), four surgeries and six doctors later, someone in the medical profession finally had enough integrity to admit defeat. It was my current gynecologist. I was 20 years old and she was telling me there was nothing more to be done short of a hysterectomy, which neither she nor I was prepared to consider.

Since I was accustomed to being rushed in and out of every doctor's office I had ever visited, I assumed this was the end of the conversation. I would now go home and concentrate on survival techniques to get me through the rest of my life. After hesitating for a moment my doctor informed me there was an alternative. I perked up, ready and willing as always to subject myself to more torture if it offered hope.

She told me about a friend of hers, a physician who has endometriosis and who had reached the same

crossroads at which I was now standing. Unwilling to
undergo a hysterectomy, which is not even a
guaranteed cure, she went elsewhere to find help and
was now feeling better than ever. I did the
obvious—asked how.

My doctor hesitated and then almost whispered the
answer as if expecting me to laugh. I was not,
however, in a position to be laughing. Seeing my
interest, she gave me the name and number of the
naturopath her friend was seeing and wished me luck.

My first appointment with the naturopath was a
shock. Prior to the visit, I received an informative
brochure that explained the principles of naturopathic
medicine, the history of it, and the education required
to become a naturopath. So I was, in that sense,
prepared. What I was not prepared for was the hour
session. After more than five years in and out of
doctors' offices in less time than it took to blink, how
could I be anything but dumbfounded? Not to
mention that a one-hour visit with the naturopath cost
the same as five minutes with any other physician who
I had seen about my endometriosis.

It has been a little more than a year since that initial
visit, but I have not forgotten it. I spent the first 45
minutes in the doctor's office (I'll call him Dr. N)
answering questions about my health. Aside from the
obvious daily pain that I associated with the
endometriosis, Dr. N talked to me about all the little
things about which I had been trying to get answers
for years. Things like why I did not have tears when I
cried, why my fingernails were full of white specks,
why I was always getting sore throats and headaches,
why I was dizzy and tired a lot, why I was continually
constipated even though I was eating a lot of fiber,
why sometimes I felt my emotions had a mind of their
own, and the list goes on. Dr. N took meticulous notes

and really seemed to believe me. For that alone, I could hardly keep from crying. Even if he could not help me, someone was finally listening to, and believing, me.

The last 15 minutes of that visit took place in an examining room. I expected the usual; clothes off, feet in the stirrups. Again I was surprised. Dr. N examined my ears, eyes, throat, tongue, glands, and reflexes, as well as the range of motion in my joints and the alignment of my spine—everything but a pelvic exam. He had reviewed my records and trusted my gynecologist's diagnosis. Dr. N drew a little blood (by now needles were *old hat*). He also gave me equipment to prepare at home for a stool sample and instructions on how to cut a piece of my hair to have it analyzed for vitamin and mineral absorption. I would send the tests to a laboratory and schedule another appointment when the results came in. This appointment would last 30 minutes, as did most of my future appointments.

The test results were presented to me as follows. The chronic pain in my abdomen was due, in part, to food allergies. I was allergic to almost all of the 100 foods for which I was tested. The most severe allergies were to wheat, dairy products, sugar, oranges, peanuts, almonds, pears, green beans, eggs and red meat. I asked what was left I could eat.

Dr. N presented me with a large packet containing a list of foods I could eat which had been compiled specifically for me. He suggested that I eliminate from my diet the foods to which I had a severe reaction, rotate every four days the foods to which I had an intermediate reaction, and rotate every other day the foods to which I reacted only moderately. The packet also contained helpful hints for planning meals, including lunch, with my specific diet in mind, eating out tips, food substitutes, and even a few recipes.

Next were the results of the mineral analysis. Basically, I was severely deficient in all of the minerals except for copper, which was high. Dr. N explained that the zinc deficiency was the cause of those white spots on my fingernails. My understanding of the reason for the deficiency is this: Because my intestines were continually subjected to foods to which I am allergic, the lining was deteriorating and unable to absorb much in the way of vitamins and minerals. Consequently, my immune system was being weakened and was now susceptible to any number of problems.

If that were not enough, I learned that on a scale of one to five (five being the worst) I had candida to the fifth degree. Apparently the *friendly* bacteria in my body had been wiped out by an overgrowth of yeast. Dr. N explained that candida caused the headaches, fatigue, and sore throats. Needless to say, I wanted to know how this happened. A number of possible causes surfaced as we talked. Previously, another doctor who did not believe my self-diagnosis of endometriosis had treated me almost monthly with antibiotics for tubal infections that probably never existed. The antibiotics were the main suspect for killing off the healthy bacteria in my body. Other contributing factors could have been birth control pills which I had taken for five years. I was prescribed the Pill for polycystic ovarian syndrome when I was 15, and I continued taking it for endometriosis. A high-sugar diet probably also contributed.

Overwhelmed and frustrated, feeling that at any moment my body was going to disintegrate, I sat and listened to Dr. N's plan of attack. Besides eliminating certain foods and rotating my diet, I would have to stay away from sweeteners, including refined sugar, maple syrup, brown sugar, corn syrup, Nutrasweet, Equal, and even foods sweetened with fruit juice.

However, I could still eat one to two servings of whole fruit a day. The yeast feeds off sugars as well as fermented products, such as alcohol, vinegar, and soy sauce, all of which I had to eliminate from my diet.

I began taking supplements to get my body back to the nutritional level of which it had fallen so short. The supplements I take include Quercetin for allergies, digestive enzymes, vitamin B6 phosphate, zinc, vitamin C, and a multiple vitamin. I was assured that by following this diet my body would heal itself naturally and would one day be ready to accommodate at least some of the restricted foods. I also took an antifungal medication to begin ridding my body of excess yeast. For the first few months, I took grapefruit seed extract and berberine Hd. Then I switched to nystatin for about six months. I also took lactobicillus acidophilus and psyllium husk powder for fiber.

When I presented this information to my family, they were not thrilled. We could not afford to feed all of us differently. My mom and brother were going to have to eat a good deal of the way I did. They would not give up wheat and dairy products, but there would be less sugar, no red meat, and many more vegetables on the daily menu.

The first few weeks of my new diet were hell. I was cranky and irritable. The sugar withdrawal was miserable, especially since I started during the holiday season. Although I was hungry and frustrated a good portion of the time, I never considered giving up. I was going to follow through with this treatment like I did with all the others and give it every opportunity to work. With this treatment, unlike the others, I was the one in control, and I did not want to let myself down the way the surgeries, drugs, and doctors had.

After a few weeks, I began to settle into my new routine. I found that many of the foods I could eat were very satisfying. These include chicken, fish, pork chops, turkey, potatoes, brown rice, and oats. I could also eat most fresh vegetables and fruit. I was eating healthier than I ever thought I had the will power to, and it felt like a major accomplishment.

After about three months, I noticed a significant decrease in my abdominal pain, headaches, and sore throat. I continued experiencing relief as long as I stayed true to the diet. My weak, peeling, and spotted nails were long, strong, clear, and pink. I had energy I had not had since I was a child. The better I felt, the easier it was to stick to my diet.

There were, of course, many times I faltered and paid for it by feeling sick. Sometimes I would give into a peanut butter sandwich or a pizza, my two biggest weaknesses, and have abdominal pain for a few days until it was out of my system. But those times come less and less these days.

I still see Dr. N every few months to maintain my improved condition and to keep the supplements at levels that will best suit my needs. He occasionally checks my eyes, ears, throat, tongue, blood pressure, and glands, but for the most part the visits consist of discussions about how I am feeling and any factors in my life that might influence my health, including on the negative side, stress at work or family tension, and on the positive side, an upcoming vacation or the prospect of a new relationship. I always leave the office feeling that I received more than my money's worth, knowing that I am welcome to call or return for anything that may arise—big or little.

Today, I feel strong and healthy. Some days I even feel invincible. And even though endometriosis is at present considered incurable, I feel cured. I feel young for the first time since I was 15 when this miserable battle began. I feel like I will live to be 100. I am not afraid of the future, and I am not afraid of dreaming. Best of all, with support and advice from Dr. N, I am in control of how I feel and that feels like the best freedom in the world.

Using Traditional Chinese Medicine to Manage Endometriosis

Eve Baron *31*
Chicago, Illinois
Diagnosed with endometriosis in 1993

I had been to five physicians within six months, and now, just two weeks before Christmas 1992, a doctor had agreed to perform a laparoscopy in January to determine if the chronic and increasing pelvic pain I was experiencing was indeed endometriosis. "What a great Christmas present," I thought. The holidays no longer looked bleak because in January the cause of this chronic pelvic pain would hopefully be discovered. I yearned to know what was wrong with me, and the anxiety that accompanied the uncertainty was taking its toll. I felt like I was living under a cloud—a dark one. I am usually an upbeat person, but every time I would feel the pain, I would get depressed. It was quite overwhelming at times. Even though I received generous emotional support from my family and friends, sometimes I would feel very alone because it was *my* pain and it was *my* body that I felt was betraying me.

It had all started the latter half of 1991. My husband and I were trying to have a second child and nothing was happening. Friends assured me that the second child frequently took longer to conceive. However, I began to notice menstrual-like cramps occurring two to three days before my period. "How strange," I thought. But I figured I just noticed the cramps because I was more in tune with my body due to the fact that I was trying to get pregnant. Then I began to have cramps during ovulation and then intermittently until I got my period.

"Now this is weird," I thought. So off to the gynecologist's office I went. Because I had an increased white blood cell count in my cervical culture, I was told I had cervicitis and was placed on an antibiotic. "I probably left a tampon in too long," I rationalized. The next month the pain returned, so I went to a family practitioner through my health maintenance organization (HMO). The second doctor proceeded to tell me about pelvic inflammatory disease. He scheduled a pelvic ultrasound, which turned out normal.

I kept going to family practitioners and gynecologists in my HMO. Every doctor stated that a fertility work-up could not be performed until we had been trying to conceive for one full year with no result. One doctor first said that I had endometriosis, and after performing an internal exam and obtaining an oral history, decided that I did not have it. He said, "In the old days we would put you to sleep and do surgery, but that costs thousands of dollars." His advice to me was to take my temperature for three months and then come back and see him.

Within that three-month time span, I found a gynecologist who suspected endometriosis and performed a diagnostic laparoscopy. I was diagnosed

with a *mild* case of endometriosis and was told that
hormone therapy was available. But it was up to me to
decide whether I wanted to keep trying to get pregnant
or to pursue drug therapy. I elected to undergo a
six-month therapy of Lupron (leuprolide acetate)
injections.

After four months on the Lupron, I noticed my
pelvic pain gradually decreasing. However, after
attending local chapter meetings of the Endometriosis
Association and talking with other women, I began to
feel uneasy about placing all my eggs in one basket,
notably the hormone therapy. I began reading about
Traditional Chinese Medicine and decided to try it. I
liked the fact that it had been around for several
thousand years and that acupuncture seemed to
stimulate the body's energy to heal itself.

It was difficult to find an acupuncturist because I
was wary of just picking one out of the telephone
book and no one I knew had ever been to one. Finally
the owner of a nearby herb store told me about a
group of Chinese doctors who exclusively practiced
acupuncture and herbal therapy. Because I am in the
medical field and work closely with physicians, I felt
more comfortable knowing that these three
acupuncturists were also licensed medical doctors. I
was extremely lucky that the practice was located only
about a mile from my home.

I started seeing the acupuncturist once every other
week. During my initial visit, he examined me by
taking my pulse on my wrist, neck, and forearm, as
well as by inspecting my tongue. He informed me that
I had a chi deficiency. Chi is translated to mean energy
in English. In addition, he said he believed that I had a
blood stasis problem in my pelvic region. He explained
that the blood in my pelvic area was not circulating

properly and that it moved sluggishly in that part of my body, becoming stagnant at times.

The acupuncturist asked me all sorts of unusual questions that no other health professional had asked, such as what were my sleeping patterns and my general emotional state. He asked questions about my diet, such as how much red meat and poultry I ate, and whether or not I avoided caffeine. I filled out a worksheet and brought it back for my next appointment. Questions on the worksheet included what was my favorite color, type of weather and season, to name a few.

During the acupuncture treatments, he placed 10 or so needles most often in my pelvic area, my legs, and my feet. Once when I was experiencing some sacral pain, he inserted needles in my sacral area and lower back. The needle insertion was very quick and most often just felt like a pin prick. After they were inserted, the doctor would twist the needles until I felt a *cramping* or *electricity* at the needle site. When I indicated that I could feel one of these sensations, he would move onto the next needle. These sensations were the most uncomfortable on my first visit. However, during subsequent sessions the sensations were less intense. After the needles were inserted, I would lie still for approximately 20 minutes in a darkened room. After the acupuncture, I always felt more relaxed.

My acupuncturist asked me if I was interested in taking Chinese herbs, and I said yes. So he gave me a bottle of liquid herbs. He told me that the bottle contained a combination of 30 different herbs, which were supposed to increase the blood flow to my pelvic area, thus eliminating the blood stagnation. I was to take the herbs two to three times daily; three times on any days that I experienced the pelvic pain. I would dissolve 30 drops at a time either in herbal tea or hot water. I was to take them preferably on an empty stomach, so I took them first thing in the morning and before I went to bed. At first I needed to dissolve the drops in herbal tea because of the peculiar odor and bitterness. But after about five weeks I was able to tolerate them in a cup of hot water.

During my treatment sessions, the acupuncturist always was very interested in my pain, my energy level, and whether I was feeling hot or cold. I noticed a decrease in my pelvic pain to the extent that I went days without a twinge of pain. My general energy level was also increasing. I hadn't realized how low my energy level had been until I noticed how much better I began to feel. As far as whether I was hot or cold, I felt I could not accurately sense my body temperature because I was still taking the Lupron and getting routine hot flashes, a common side effect. Generally though, I was usually cold and I love hot weather.

After two acupuncture treatments plus daily herbs, my pelvic pain was 99% improved.

I also noticed an improvement in two incisions from my laparoscopy which had healed poorly. Four months after surgery, the umbilical incision still had bruising around it, and the incision above the pubic bone was red, raised, and hard—almost scablike. After two acupuncture treatments and herbs, the bruising disappeared from the incision and the other scar was flat, smooth, and no longer red.

After my sixth injection of Lupron, I began to experience intense anxiety, with incidents of insomnia and depression. My eyes started twitching, and one day I woke up and my mouth was twitching. I panicked and was sure that something terrible was happening to me. I called Tapp Pharmaceuticals, the maker of Lupron. A manufacturer's representative told me that no one had ever reported "twitching" as a side effect. I contacted my HMO and was able to see a family practitioner that day. The doctor examined me and said that there was nothing wrong with me except that I was "majorly stressed out." I felt relieved with the doctor's assessment of my twitching; at least it was not a symptom of a new problem. But deep down I suspected that the intense feelings of anxiety and sleeplessness were manifesting themselves in the physical side effect of twitching. I believed that the Lupron was the culprit behind all three.

At my next acupuncture treatment, I told the acupuncturist the extent of my stress and anxiety. He stated that my pulses indicated that I was feeling a great deal of stress. So he incorporated acupuncture points into my treatment to calm me and reduce my feelings of anxiety. Although the relief from my anxiety was temporary, lasting only until the next day, it felt great to catch a glimpse of my old self. My feelings of extreme anxiety, the insomnia, and the depression continued but gradually lessened until six or eight weeks after my last Lupron injection. The twitching gradually decreased and stopped about five weeks after the last injection.

Around this time, I was weighing the pros and cons of taking Clomid to begin ovulating if my period did not return on its own within six weeks of completing the Lupron shots. One HMO gynecologist, who was not my regular doctor and whom I saw only briefly, highly recommended this course of treatment. However, the thought of another powerful drug in my system was not appealing to me. This particular physician also wrote me a prescription for a pain reliever because I had such a "terrible disease" that I would undoubtedly need this prescription in the future. "Nice positive thinking," I thought, and vowed

I would not get the prescription filled. Fortunately, I had never needed prescription-strength pain relievers before, and after the hormone therapy I naturally thought that I would feel better, not worse. The fact that this doctor never bothered to ask me about my previous history regarding endometriosis, except for the infertility, really irritated me. His fatalistic attitude regarding the chronicity of endometriosis angered me and reaffirmed my inclination toward alternative therapies, especially Traditional Chinese Medicine.

I discussed the Clomid option with the acupuncturist. He was candid about the fact that he thought it was unwise. The acupuncturist believed that my pituitary gland would not know whether it was coming or going, after being in pseudo-menopause for six months with the Lupron and then being jumpstarted to ovulate with the Clomid. He suggested trying to stimulate the pituitary gland using acupuncture. Two months after my last Lupron injection and thirteen days following the acupuncture treatment session, I got my period.

I had some menstrual cramps the first two days, but over-the-counter pain relievers did the job. I took the Chinese herbs three times a day during my period. The days that I did have cramps, the herbs relieved them for two to three hours after I took them.

At my next acupuncture appointment, I discussed with the acupuncturist my fear of being unable to get pregnant again. In addition to addressing the blood stasis problem in my pelvis, he placed needles in acupuncture points to stimulate fertility. I do not remember where the needles were placed for the fertility treatments, but there were twice as many needles in me than I ever had before.

Two weeks later I had a positive pregnancy test. I contacted the acupuncturist immediately. He advised me to cease taking the herbs and to discontinue the acupuncture treatments. However, he indicated that acupuncture could assist in alleviating any adverse pregnancy symptoms, such as nausea and carpal tunnel syndrome.

Around the same time I began acupuncture, I also did two other lifestyle changes that I believe contributed to the elimination of my pain and my ability to conceive.

For one, I started doing yoga. I bought a videotape and performed yoga approximately 30 minutes daily. I chose yoga basically because I could work with the tape while my son was napping. Because it is quiet I did not have to worry about waking him. The yoga made me feel relaxed and refreshed immediately afterward. During my high-anxiety episode, I really noticed a lessening in my anxiousness for at least an hour or two after doing the yoga.

Second, I began eating more organic foods. I started to eat only organic poultry and red meat. In addition, much of the fruits and vegetables I consumed were also organic. My husband worked near an organic food store with a large selection, so we had easy access to these goods. I also started attempting to eliminate dairy products from my diet and to increase my water intake.

I made these dietary changes after discussing my diet with the acupuncturist and after hearing a homeopath and chiropractor internist speak at separate meetings of the local Endometriosis Association chapter. The latter strongly advised against eating any non-organic poultry or red meat because of the hormones that the animals consume. I thought that made sense. And here I was on a drug for six months that was trying to lessen my estrogen, while the meat I was eating most likely had been exposed to an unnatural amount of hormones, notably estrogen.

My experience with Traditional Chinese Medicine was very positive. I truly believe that it can benefit women with endometriosis. The yoga and dietary changes were also beneficial. Perhaps it was the combination of these interventions that decreased my pain and helped me to conceive. No one can know for sure. However, I do know that if ever my endometriosis surfaces again, Traditional Chinese Medicine will most definitely be part of my treatment program.

Putting Homeopathy to the Test

Barbara Bornmann *30s*
Brooklyn, New York
Diagnosed with endometriosis in 1988

My homeopath put two small pellets in an eyedropper
bottle filled with water and vodka. He shook it
vigorously ten times, and the undissolved pellets sunk
to the bottom. "From the moment the pellets hit the
water, the entire contents of this bottle became your
remedy," he said. I sat there looking at this bottle
thinking, "You've got to be kidding."

For the past two hours we had discussed the sum
total of my life: childhood diseases, chronic problems,
hereditary health of my immediate and extended
family, family dynamics, sex life, emotional life,
psychological life, spiritual life, intellectual pursuits,
compulsions, addictions, and my favorite colors. His
recommendations for my first remedy and emotional
counseling were made based on this first session.

The homeopath told me to take a couple of drops
on or under my tongue twice a day. He cautioned me
to be careful not to touch the dropper to my mouth or
it would become contaminated. He asked me to take

the remedy immediately so he could see my response. I put a couple of drops carefully on my tongue. I felt a sort of dizziness like something awakened in my head. He told me that I had a good response, and I left.

Let me explain exactly where I was in proximity to my laparoscopy, which turned into a laparotomy, for severe Stage IV endometriosis on January 28, 1988. My decision following surgery was to start hormone treatment along with nutritional changes. I declined additional laser surgery. I took Danocrine (danazol) for almost three months, but called it quits when I awoke out of a sound sleep screaming—male hormones can do that to you. There was no circulation in my left leg, and I hobbled about until it returned. I then had a shot of Depo-Provera, which resulted in frequent and acausal bleeding. After three months, my surgeon suggested a mega-dose shot of Depo-Provera to stop the bleeding and to stop my body from trying to menstruate. That left me face down for 36 hours. Luckily, my family was around to take care of me. Eight months after surgery, I went on a low-dose birth control pill, a choice I had been trying to avoid because of the correlation between high estrogen and breast cancer.

It was May 21, 1990, twenty months since I had started the Pill. The Pill regulated my body with remarkable precision. My body fell into a 30-day cycle and stayed there. I bled a small amount and could accurately predict the time and length of my periods.

As theories surfaced that endometriosis may be aggravated by excessive estrogen, I became more and more uncomfortable with the Pill. I felt trapped by the medical model, to which I had given my power, so I sought an alternative approach.

I gravitated to homeopathy because my grandfather's brother was a homeopath who treated

my father's family for ailments. It represented a
paradigm I could trust. I chose a homeopath who was
not an M.D., but was a seasoned and intuitive lay
practitioner. I wanted someone who could work with
me intuitively because I felt that my endometriosis was
not only caused by the physical imbalances from
hereditary tendencies, environmental toxins, and a
weakened immune system, but was supported by an
underlying psychological/emotional/spiritual
imbalance. How I responded to my physical
imbalances, such as avoidance behavior, addictive or
self-destructive creative patterns, emotional upsets or
lack of spiritual intregration and direction, was an
equal cause. There was also a severe imbalance in the
masculine and feminine energies of my nature. I was
very masculine and denied my feminine energies.

   Listening to the radio program *Natural Living* on
WBAI radio NY, I heard the voice of a dynamic healer
who was going to be teaching a course on nutrition for
immune system deficiency disorders. I took the course
and when she was absent for one of the sessions she
sent her husband, a homeopath, as a substitute to talk
about homeopathy. As fate would have it, I found my
seasoned and intuitive lay practitioner.

   Homeopathy, introduced in 1810 by Samuel
Hahnemann, is based on the science of
homotoxicology, which has two major phases in the
progression of disease. The *humoral phase*, in which
the body can heal itself, and the *cellular phase*, in
which the body requires serious medical intervention.
It seems that the entire medical establishment in
America would have women believe that
endometriosis, along with cancer, is in the cellular
phase. This is incorrect. The fact is that endometriosis
is in the humoral phase and is a disease that can be

helped dramatically by rebalancing the homeostatis of the body.

I've come to understand homeopathy as a process likened to peeling away the layers of an onion. The remedies are always digging at, and exposing, imbalances, and the emotional response is a natural occurrence in this process. To illustrate what I mean by an *emotional response*, I will use an example of one of my remedies, gynacoheel, as defined in *Ordinato Antihomotoxica et Materia Medica*, the bible of homeopathy. Gynacoheel is made up of 11 constituents (elements) of which 3 have emotional indications (conditions it treats). One of the constituents is *Apis mellifica* (honey bee), which has indications listed as edema, ovaritis, hypersensitivity, and nervousness. As a result of taking the remedy, I became extremely hypersensitive and nervous for a period of time, which was emotionally upsetting. As my body worked back to a time when I was in balance, adverse symptoms and reactions occurred. Deep issues of self-acceptance, self-love, and self-esteem also surfaced. For support, which was necessary at that time, I kept a journal and began seeing a therapist. Homeopathy teaches us to accept our physical symptoms, feel them and let them go, instead of suppressing or controlling them.

The success of homeopathic medicine depends upon the patient's ability to help herself in all areas of holistic health and share intuitive information in uncovering the different imbalances that led to the disease. Apart from helping me assert control over my body, homeopathy has allowed me to unravel the patterns and process that led to the disease in the first place. Homeopathy is contrary to the *wonder pill* approach to medicine so widely accepted in America where the patient has no involvement or responsibility in the process of healing.

From the moment that first drop of homeopathic remedy hit my tongue, a war raged inside, between the part of me that believes in the medical establishment and the part of me that believes in myself. I could feel the patriarchal bias of the medical establishment implementing treatments for endometriosis that manipulate and control women. Personally, I was too uncomfortable with the feeling of being a guinea pig to test hormone treatments for which there were no long-term studies. I had to learn to trust myself and the power of my body to heal itself.

When my homeopath suggested that I stop taking the birth control pill, I resisted. We decided I would continue taking the Pill until I felt comfortable stopping. This meant I would be taking the Pill and the homeopathic remedy at the same time with the goal of eliminating the Pill.

The first day I took the remedy I felt something changing but had no idea what. By the second day I was feeling irritable and my body was starting to cramp. I thought this was odd because it was mid-cycle during ovulation. By the third day I was cramping and spotting, and by the fourth day I started to bleed.

I called the homeopath in near hysteria because the goal was to stop my excessive bleeding. He told me that the remedy was also an antidote for the birth control pill. That ridiculous eyedropper full of what appeared to be nothing was actually knocking the Pill out of my system. I was impressed. I was also hooked. We cut back on the remedy, and within six months I was able to stop taking the Pill. This was an incredibly difficult time. My body was confused and I was experiencing exacerbated symptoms, but I was determined to get off the Pill.

Before you embark on this path, it is important to know that homeopathy actually brings out symptoms. When I started taking the homeopathic remedies, my symptoms became more severe than they had been in the past.

My symptoms were weakness, sore throat, headaches, chronic fatigue, an aching pain in the lungs prior to my period, swelling and burning due to vaginitis, bloating, and a skin condition on my face and eyelids. The skin condition was diagnosed as Acne Rosacea by a dermatologist and as a yeast condition by a holistic medical doctor. The dermatologist recommended antibiotics, which are not part of a holistic protocol. This skin problem could also have been due to homeopathic healing; as the endometriosis heals, the body eliminates the disease through lesions or boils on the skin. I sometimes had a feeling of being overwhelmed—not by exhaustion—but as if I was out of control. As far as pelvic pain goes, I had general dull abdominal pain (which rose and fell with the tide of my menstrual cycle), gas pain, localized stabbing pain in the left or right wall of my uterus, nausea, and aching stomach pain.

My symptoms became so severe when I was first taking the remedy that I had myself tested for sexually-transmitted diseases and viruses as possible co-factors contributing to my weakened state. Blood tests and vaginal cultures revealed that my immune system was compromised by Epstein-Barr, herpes I, cytomegalovirus, and at one point, candida and streptococcus B. I was given another remedy to address these symptoms at subsequent visits to the homeopath.

Gradually my symptoms lessened as my immune system strengthened and my body struggled to balance. For example, one month I would have strong period cramps on the first day. Another month I would have vaginitis before my period. The next month I would have pain when I ovulated, along with elevated estrogen levels. (I know when my estrogen is high because I get nauseous, intense headaches, breast tenderness, and a feeling of fullness throughout my body.) Each month, the different symptoms were isolated, which indicated that my body was balancing. The homeopath explained that the remedy stimulates the body's own defenses to heal itself.

From the time I reached puberty until my surgery for endometriosis, I always had one week of premenstrual syndrome and long periods characterized by heavy bleeding. The results from my homeopathic program have been staggering. Nowadays, my hard-earned balance affords me a two-day period with cramps issuing between a one- to six-hour warning and sometimes no warning and no cramps. My homeopath also encouraged me to stop taking ibuprofen for the cramping because it is an unnatural substance that the body cannot metabolize. Regular Bayer aspirin was recommended and I recently checked my bottle to find that I have only taken nine aspirin in three years. Ironically, I have very little unmanagable pain.

The following is a list of homeopathic remedies taken over a period of three years. I made two or three visits to the homeopath per year. At the first visit he recommended sepia as the remedy; the second visit, gynacoheel and BHI inflammation, and so on. Each individual would have a program unique to her. The only remedy specifically for endometriosis is gynacoheel. This is not a recommendation, but for informational purposes only. What is important to note is how many systems of the body are being treated.

Sepia 6c

Purpose: Constitutional remedy to treat the endometriosis and the immune system.

Dosage: Three times a day the first week, twice a day the second week, stabilizing at once a day every week for four months.

Gyanocoheel

Purpose: To treat ovarian cysts and endometriosis.

Dosage: Once a day for three months.

BHI Inflammation

Purpose: To treat Streptococcus B.

Dosage: Once a day for two months.

Hormeel

Purpose: To balance hormones and the endocrine system.

Dosage: Twice a day for one month.

Psoronoheel

Purpose: Deeper constitutional remedy to treat chronic disease.

Dosage: Once a week alternating with Glyoxl.

Glyoxl

Purpose: To boost the immune system.

Dosage: Once a week alternating with Psoronoheel.

Lymphomyocot

Purpose: To cleanse the lymphatic system.

Dosage: Once a day for three months.

Argentum Nitricum 6c

Purpose: To treat current symptoms and weaknesses associated with endometriosis and other life patterns.

Dosage: Once a day for a month.

Engystol

Purpose: To reduce the Epstein-Barr titer.
Dosage: Once a week before bed.

Glyola

Purpose: To enhance cell respiration.
Dosage: One dose (several pellets) once a week for three weeks.

Ubichinon

Purpose: To enhance cell enzyme activity.
Dosage: Twice a week for one month.

Argentum Nitircum 30c

Purpose: To expose and treat deep childhood patterns. For example, one of the indications of this remedy is a "fear of being alone." I was terrified of being alone as a child.
Dosage: One dose (several pellets) every six months.

In contrast to the above program with my lay homeopath, I recently started a program with a holistic medical doctor who works with homeopathy, nutrition, and supplements. He uses applied kinesiology, a chiropractic form of treatment that uses muscle testing as a diagnostic tool, to test the body for weaknesses. The testing confirmed weaknesses in my immune, digestive, endocrine, and hepatic systems, revealing specific vitamin deficiencies and a pool of underlying viral activity. This program's purpose is to aggressively target these symptoms, not to deal with other levels of well-being. If my homeopathic journey had started with this type of program, I might have dismissed or overlooked the emotional, spiritual, and deep constitutional problems associated with my endometriosis.

The reason that I have been successful with homeopathy is because I was willing to make lifestyle changes and because I have worked synergistically with other holistic therapies including nutrition, supplements, vitamins, exercise, meditation, rest, yoga, magnetic therapy, shiatsu, jin shin jyutsu, as well as emotional and spiritual counseling.

I would like to briefly discuss nutrition because it played an important role in the success of my homeopathic healing. After surgery I began the process of re-evaluating my diet by eliminating all caffeine, salt, sugar, and alcohol. I wanted to be well more than anything in the world, so I started to learn about holistic health and nutrition. The big obstacle for me was dairy products; it took me two years to eliminate dairy. My diet is now primarily a nondairy, high-fiber, low-fat, low-protein, vegetarian diet with seasonal fish. It has been proven that vegetarian women have lower levels of estrogen than non-vegetarian women, according to Dr. Christiane Northrup. In her audiotape *Honoring Our Bodies—Endometriosis*, she suggests using diet as a first step to reducing estrogen levels, assuming that high-circulating estrogen is part of the problem. Foods that may contribute to high estrogen levels include meat, milk, eggs, dairy products, alcohol, and foods containing yeast.

The fact that endometriosis was not surgically removed from my stomach, intestines, and other delicate organs turned out to be a blessing in disguise. By accident, I learned that much of my pain was directly related to what I ate. Those really terrific cold sesame noodles would leave me cramped and in tears by 3 A.M. In disbelief, I ate them again with the same results. Hence, I developed the *cold sesame noodle test* to measure the progress of my endometriosis treatment.

My dynamic teacher once said, "You're only as healthy as you can digest, assimilate, and eliminate. A healthy digestive tract produces one to three bowel movements a day." It is a known fact that a high fiber, vegetarian diet will keep the digestive tract optimumly well. Furthermore, I am certain this diet has affected my cholesterol, which is 125.

My local health food store, and now a neighborhood food co-op, keeps me in organic vegetables. These include onions, garlic, broccoli, carrots, beans, asparagus, beets, white and sweet potatos, acorn, kaboocha and butternut squash, zuchinni, tomatoes, eggplant, regular and shiitake mushrooms, kale, collards, spinach, sprouts, and lettuce greens. I also enjoy sea vegetables such as nori, hijiki, and arame.

For carbohydrates, I eat soba noodles, artichoke and semolina pasta, brown rice, barley, quinoa, millet, cous cous, tortillas and non-yeasted breads. Because the body is 15 percent to 20 percent protein, I eat a corresponding proportion of protein in my diet. For protein, I eat a variety of legumes and beans, tempeh, tofu, sardines in water, white fish, soy milk, soy cheese, and soy yogurt. I eat oatmeal as well as oat bran and five-grain cereals. Fruits I consume include bananas, apples, grapefruits, oranges, pears, melons, and avocados. I drink fresh carrot, celery, cucumber, and beet juice. I like macrobiotic, Japanese, Italian, Mexican, and Indian foods.

When I shared my health program with my surgeon, her response was, "What *do* you eat? Well, whatever you're doing Barb, just keep doing it."

The following are the supplements I use:

➢ Vitamin A—25,000 IU daily
➢ All B's—100 mg daily (orally), up to 3,000 (intravenously)
➢ Pantothenic acid—100 mg three times a day
➢ Vitamin C—3,000 to 18,000 mg daily (orally), up to 75,000 mg (intravenously)

> Vitamin E—400 IU daily
> Borage oil—One capsule a day (Instead of using evening primrose oil, I take borage oil which has six times as much gamma-linolenic acid and is less expensive. Because of their high content of this acid, these oils inhibit prostaglandin activity.)
> Calcium—1,000 mg daily
> Magnesium—400 mg daily
> Kelp—Two to six pills a day
> Wellness multiple or other natural multiple vitamin
> Pro-gest cream—A natural progesterone to rub into my abdomen for premenstrual syndrome symptoms and hormone balance

Detoxification was a necessary part of changing my diet. I used various detoxification products for one to two months at a time, according to how I felt. This includes aloe vera which I take daily because of its wonderful healing properties. I learned to listen to the integrity of the body—my body knows when to take them just like it knows when my estrogen is skyrocketing. Products I have used include the following:

> Chlorophyll products to nourish and cleanse the blood: Green Magma, Sun Chlorella, Wheat Grass, liquid chlorophyll
> Hydrogen peroxide to oxygenate the blood: Dr. Donsbach Superoxy Plus
> Friendly bacteria to promote intestinal balance: Flora Balance, acidophilus
> Grapefruit seed extract to rid the body of micro-organisms and yeast: Citricidal, Paramicrocydin, caprillic acid
> Milk thistle to promote healthy liver function: Silymarin, Thisilyn

➤ Anti-viral products: Monolaurin, lomation root, garlic
➤ Detoxification products to rid the body of metabollic waste: Cell Guard
➤ Fiber to keep the colon cleansed: psyllium, Triphala (3 Indian herbs)
➤ To increase energy and vitality: Co Q10
➤ To increase cellular metabolism: Germanium

I also use herbs including don quai, red raspberry, siberian ginseng, ginkgo biloba, cell tea, black cohosh, ginger root, dandelion, echinacea, pau d'arco, chaparral, detox tea, herbal eye wash, myrrh, slippery elm and valerian root. I use herbs primarily in a liquid form. I either take a couple of drops on my tongue or put a few drops in herbal tea. Occasionally I will use herbs in pill form if they are available. I buy these herbs either from my homeopath or from the health food store. I use filtered water to make these teas and also to drink and cook with.

My lifestyle includes routine saunas or very hot baths, aerobic activity, and colonics, all of which are great for detoxification and maintenance. Saunas allow the body temperature to rise, which inhibits viral activity, thus eliminating toxins through the skin. Aerobic exercise also allows the body to sweat and increases circulation and respiration. I try to sweat at least four times a week. I feel colonics are a necessary part of ridding the body of accumulated waste. Believe me, when you see what looks like petrified wood come out of your body you will know what I mean. Looking at a cross-section drawing of the colon, it is obvious that there are many places for toxins to hide. A colonic is given by a therapist and I would recommend disposable equipment and filtered water.

In closing, I would like to honor the teachers and holistic health professionals who have supported me on my path to wellness. My journey of almost six years has been from severe Stage IV endometriosis to a physical state where my endometriosis is not recurring. I am the most balanced and healthy that I have been in my life! The protocol outlined here has allowed me both to heal and co-exist with the endometriosis still present from surgery. I've learned from my endometriosis, for it has an elusive integrity that exceeds human understanding and scientific limitations.

As I look back on my life I realize that this new balance is profound. Life is worth living to the fullest. I hope that every woman facing the endometriosis challenge is able to find balance within her life. For me, the key was finding it deep within—that connection to nature and my spiritual connection to the universe—instead of something outside of myself to heal or make me whole.

A Long Road to Pain Relief

Ruth Carol *29*
Skokie, Illinois
Diagnosed with endometriosis in 1983

I had my first period when I was exactly 12½ years old. I woke up in the middle of the night with terrible cramps. I thought I had stomach cramps from something I ate for dinner. The heating pad brought no relief. I tossed and turned for hours trying to make the pain go away. Then I got my period.

I spent the next six and one-half years going to doctors to find out why my periods were so painful, consisted of such a heavy flow, and came increasingly closer together. The pain would typically start with the onset of my period and would last throughout it. The pain ranged from stabs and cramps to dull aches and pulling sensations. Over the years, my cycles gradually shrank from 28 days to 14. The gynecologists just said I had painful periods; after all, my mother did too. They prescribed painkillers, everything from Ponstel and Naprosyn to Motrin (which the doctors think ate a hole in my colon) and Percodan (a synthetic codeine). The pain was often unbearable. Until the painkillers kicked in, I would sometimes just sit with the heating pad turned on high and cry in despair.

Finally the twelfth or so gynecologist I saw suggested my pain could be caused by endometriosis. He performed a diagnostic laparoscopy (laser surgery was nonexistent at that time), and the diagnosis was confirmed. I was diagnosed with mild endometriosis at age 19. I was prescribed the birth control pill, which I took for six years. It brought total relief for a few years and then gradually the pain returned.

In 1987 I had a laser laparoscopy with a reproductive endocrinologist who was highly recommended. My gynecologist had relocated out of state. The diagnosis remained the same, the prognosis good; all the endometriosis was lasered out. I continued on the Pill. The surgery bought a symptom-free year, but the pain gradually returned. Eighteen months later I was close to my pre-surgery pain levels, downing a minimum of six painkillers each day of my period.

I made an appointment with the reproductive endocrinologist to tell him about the recurring symptoms. He said that many women experience a recurrence of the symptoms approximately two years after laser surgery and some opt to have the surgery biannually as a maintenance plan. The other option was Lupron, which was still considered an experimental drug at the time. I was concerned about the lack of long-term studies, so I declined taking it. At that point I decided there must be a better way to treat my endometriosis.

By then, I had been married a few years, and my husband and I decided to try and start a family. We anticipated having problems because of the endometriosis, so we figured this was as good a time as any to start. When I stopped taking the Pill, the pain got worse. I began experiencing cramps not only when I menstruated but when I ovulated as well. Between ovulation and the onset of my period, I had bouts of constipation and diarrhea.

Around that time a friend told me that her gynecologist recommended taking evening primrose oil to relieve her severe premenstrual syndrome and that her symptoms had diminished significantly from doing so. I remember having read somewhere about studies on the use of evening primrose oil in relieving endometriosis cramps. Thus began my research into alternative therapies for endometriosis. I read everything I could find on evening primrose oil. This lead me to research vitamin therapy and nutrition. There was not much information available, as is still the case.

Based on the information I gathered, I self-prescribed a daily vitamin regimen consisting of a high B-complex vitamin, vitamins A (beta carotene), C, and E, and evening primrose oil. I also made sure to get vitamins with selenium, magnesium, and zinc. I experimented with different vitamins and other supplements for several months. I used the book *Vitamin Bible* by Earl Mindell to make sure I was not taking toxic amounts of vitamins and also that I was not using vitamins in amounts that would cancel each other out. I purchased the vitamins from a health food store and a discount mail order catalog.

I tried making only one change at a time and keeping up with it for three months at a time to objectively evaluate how effective each therapy was. For example, I took chlorophyll, which relieved some of my bowel symptoms. But then I read more about candida and thought maybe that could be a contributing problem, given my cyclical bowel upsets. So I began taking lactobacillus acidophilus, which is supposed to maintain normal intestinal flora. I found it to be more effective than the chlorophyll. Of course, that prompted me to investigate whether I had an overgrowth of yeast as do many women with endometriosis. So I went to an allergist to get tested for candida, but it turned out that my yeast levels were normal.

I noticed an improvement after one month of taking evening primrose oil. I was skeptical, thinking maybe it was the power of suggestion; however, after taking it for three months I noticed a significant decrease in the pain I experienced during my periods. The vitamins seemed responsible for supplying me with an abundance of energy.

Although I had read about the importance of diet in treating endometriosis, I did not make too many changes in mine. For several years, I had not eaten red meat or any form of caffeine, including coffee, non-herbal tea, carbonated beverages, and chocolate. I also made a conscious effort to avoid high-sugar foods. I ate a lot of vegetables and complex carbohydrates. I also exercised three times a week.

Around this time I became acquainted with an acupuncturist who had become intrigued with endometriosis because of his work with patients who had other chronic diseases.

In researching acupuncture, I learned of the philosophy behind Traditional Chinese Medicine. Essentially, the goal of Traditional Chinese Medicine is to create a balance in the body. It views the body as one system that must be treated as a whole, contrary to Western medicine which isolates whatever is the problem and then treats it. In Traditional Chinese Medicine, organs cannot be treated in isolation because what affects one affects them all. This philosophy made sense to me.

At that time I was seeing a different reproductive endocrinologist. Because I was trying to conceive, we were trying to determine whether I ovulated on a regular basis. Through blood tests and ultrasounds, which are routine for fertility workups, we learned that I ovulated on my own, but that I had a luteal phase defect—which meant that the last half of my cycle, from ovulation to the onset of my period, was shorter than the first half of my cycle. As a result, I was producing low levels of progesterone, which is needed in abundance for a fertilized egg to implant in the uterus. This is common for women with endometriosis, but it meant that even if I conceived the egg would likely be unable to implant, resulting in a miscarriage.

The doctor suggested either taking fertility drugs or progesterone suppositories to beef up my hormone levels. I opted for the second choice because I knew that I was ovulating, so I did not need or want the excess estrogen in my system from the drugs to wreak havoc on my endometriosis. The doctor said he would be happy if we could raise my progesterone to at least 10 micrograms per liter, but 11 or 12 micrograms per liter would be preferable.

Then I got the idea that I could use acupuncture to treat the endometriosis and balance my hormone levels. At least it was worth a try. The acupuncturist I befriended was amenable to trying this, even though he had never done anything like it. He explained that he would diagnose me using Traditional Chinese Medicine and would not treat me to raise my progesterone levels, per se, but that that should be an outcome of balancing my hormonal system. He diagnosed me by observing my tongue, taking my pulses, and asking several questions about the pain I had and even my lifestyle, including my exercise regimen and eating habits. I was diagnosed as having a blood stagnation and chi deficiency.

I saw the acupuncturist once a week for a couple of months, and then once every two weeks, usually right before ovulation and the onset of my period. During the acupuncture sessions, he placed approximately ten needles, usually in my feet or below the knee. On occasion he would put a needle in my hand, head, ear, or around my belly button, depending on the particular set of symptoms we were working on for that session. I could barely feel the needles being inserted, but I could often tell what organ he was working on because that area would develop a minor, dull ache. When he twisted the needles to stimulate the points, I felt a brief sensation, but it was not what I would describe as painful, just uncomfortable. I would lie still on the acupuncture table in the darkened room listening to New Age music for about twenty minutes. As part of the treatment, I took dong quai and various other herbs to detoxify and strengthen my system. The dong quai was a liquid, and the herbs were in pill form.

Two odd things happened to me when I started Traditional Chinese Medicine. The first thing was one morning after a session I woke up with little red, scaly dots on my chest and stomach. This had happened to me once before shortly before being diagnosed with endometriosis. At that time, I went to a dermatologist to get rid of the unexplained skin condition. It was such a peculiar thing that I never forgot what those patches looked like. The second thing was after another session my face swelled up along the bridge of my nose and my eyes were all puffy. Again, this had happened to me shortly before being diagnosed and had prompted one gynecologist to think I was allergic to my hormones because this occurred before the onset of my period for several months. At that time, I had to

take medicine to reduce the swelling. Once I went on
the Pill, it did not recur. Both times I called the
acupuncturist to tell him about these incidents and he
said that it was my body getting rid of the
endometriosis. I was skeptical, but also impressed.
After a few months of acupuncture, my periods were
lighter and shorter. I was now taking only two
Anaprox with the onset of my period.

I also began documenting the results of the blood
tests to determine my progesterone levels. Prior to my
acupuncture treatments, the average progesterone level
was 6.5 micrograms per liter. After the acupuncture,
the average progesterone level was 11.9 micrograms
per liter. The doctor seemed surprised by the sudden
increase in progesterone. I told him he would not
believe it if I told him how I did it, so he was better off
not asking. He just said to keep *it* up, whatever *it* was.
I had documented the tests for seven months. On the
last acupuncture treatment, the acupuncturist also
placed needles in some points for fertility. I got
pregnant the following month and discontinued the
herbs and acupuncture treatments.

Unfortunately I had a miscarriage when I was four
months pregnant. It was not a complete shock because
from the beginning my HCG (human chorionic
gonadotropin, commonly referred to as the pregnancy
hormone) levels were irratic, and the doctor warned us
that a miscarriage was a distinct possibility.

During an emergency D&C (dilation & curettage),
the attending physician punctured my uterus and
sucked out 20 inches of my bowel, which he had
mistaken for fetal tissue. A colorectal surgeon had to
repair the bowel, and my reproductive endocrinologist
came in to repair the uterus. I was in the hospital for
one week recovering from bowel surgery and a
laparotomy, and spent another two months recovering

at home. Ironically, following the surgery I had more problems with my bowel than I did the endometriosis. Luckily I found a gastroenterologist who prescribed medication that I still take for my bowel. I also get B-12 shots four times a year. I now have what the doctors call short bowel syndrome.

A few months later I was back at the acupuncturist to get my whole *female* system in balance. The endometriosis pain had gotten a little worse: I now had one day of discomfort with the onset of my period. But I was unsure which was the culprit: the endometriosis, my body still recovering from the miscarriage, or the surgery, or a combination thereof. Either way, I did not want to lose the gains I had made using the vitamins, evening primrose oil, and acupuncture. I figured the four period-free months I gained with the pregnancy were cancelled out by the shock my system received from the miscarriage and surgery. So I was starting anew.

My acupuncturist was now treating several women with endometriosis and was even participating in a private research project studying traditional Chinese herb formulas in treating dysmenorrhea in endometriosis patients. I agreed to participate. After one month of taking the herbs, I got pregnant again and had to drop out of the study.

This time, I had an uneventful pregnancy and a precious baby girl. I breastfed her exclusively until she was 9½ months old. As of this writing, she is 14 months old, I still breastfeed her (although much less frequently now), and I have had only four periods. I have had minor discomfort. For the last two periods, instead of reaching for the painkillers I drank raspberry leaf tea to relieve the cramps. Once my period resumes on a regular basis, I plan to return to the acupuncturist. I still take the vitamins and evening primrose oil daily.

I recently began seeing a homeopath to help heal my bowel. Although the medication keeps the symptoms in check, I prefer fixing the underlying problem. But of course, as any holistic practitioner would do, the homeopath is working with me to heal my *whole* system, including my bowel and female organs.

Is Your Body Toxic?

Carolyn Levine Cohen *42*
Atlanta, Georgia
Diagnosed with endometriosis in 1979

I was diagnosed with endometriosis in 1979 and was told the usual medical shpiel . . . "We don't know why you have it or what causes it." One explanation was that I was a working woman and had not yet had children. After all, endometriosis was dubbed *the working woman's syndrome.*

The treatment of choice back then was birth control pills. I was a little reluctant to go back on the Pill because of the previous side effects I had experienced in my early twenties. However, I was experiencing so much pain during my periods, I was game to try anything. I was lucky and the Pill put the endometriosis in remission. Then I tried Danocrine (danazol) for a short time, but it gave me migraine headaches. So I went back on the Pill and did fine until 1986. At that time my gynecologist said that I had been on the Pill too long and it was unwise to keep a woman my age (35 at the time) on the Pill. Needless to say I was a bit nervous going off it for fear the pain would return. But I eventually stopped and did fine for about one and one-half years.

Then in 1987 my husband and I bought a house that had a natural gas leak in it. This pushed my immune system over the edge. I became allergic to everything in my environment. And once again the endometriosis got out of control.

One of the worst symptoms I developed from my highly allergic state was an uncontrollable cough that lasted between two and three hours at a time and would occur two to three times a day. Had endometrosis attacked my lungs? The doctors did not know. We had scheduled laser surgery three times. But each time I had to cancel it because I was too "reactive" to even go into the hospital, let alone a surgery suite. The oxygen level in my blood was low, and nobody could tell me why! My whole body was going out of control, and the medical profession I had worked in for 15 years was failing me.

Finally, I found my way to a clinic for the chemically sensitive in Dallas. There I learned about the toxins in our environment, homes, and bodies. I also learned through the other patients about acupuncture, homeopathy, and herbs, to name a few.

When I left the clinic, my first step was to start cleaning up the toxins in my house and my body. In situations like mine, nothing can be accomplished overnight. I had 38 years of polluting my body with the foods I ate, the water I drank, and the air I breathed.

The first thing I did was to pull up the new carpet that was filling the air I breathed with formaldehyde, glues, and gasses, all of which were toxic to me. We made my bedroom "safe" by enclosing the mattress in a non-treated cotton encasement and using only all-cotton sheets, pillows, and blankets. The furniture was all mostly old, so that could stay because all of the chemical smells from the materials used to make it had significantly decreased. We also bought an air machine to eliminate dust, molds, and chemicals. The theory behind making the bedroom as pure and clean as possible is this: Our bodies heal while we sleep. The fewer the toxins, such as dyes, sprays, petrochemicals, and pollutants, we are exposed to while we sleep, the more chance the toxins that accumulated in our bodies during the day can be eliminated and repair work on damaged organs, tissues, and cells can be expedited.

The next step was cleaning up the rest of the house. We got rid of all the household cleaning chemicals underneath the sink. We managed to fill two garbage cans with all of these toxic chemicals that our wonderful bodies automatically eliminate from our system to keep us relatively healthy. It is amazing how many poisons we have just lying around our homes that we are unaware of.

Next was cleaning up my diet. I started eating whole grain foods such as brown rice, quinoa, millet, and buckwheat. These are foods that are not chemically processed and have higher concentrations of nutrients. Also, I started buying organic beef and chicken. *Organic* foods are those that have not been treated with any pesticides, herbicides, hormones, antibiotics, or preservatives. I started eating more vegetables, organic ones whenever possible. I began drinking filtered water, too.

But I soon learned that just because I was eating healthier did not mean that I was digesting properly. When eating I could feel a gurgle in my throat, which indicated to me that I needed something to help break down my foods.

I sought a chiropractor because intuitively I knew if I was aligned, I could heal. My chiropractor used a technique called clinical kinesiology. With this method, he used muscle testing to find out whether a particular substance, such as a supplement, a food, a place, or even an activity, was strengthening or weakening my body's meridians. Placing a vitamin C, for example, on my stomach meridian, the chiropractor would apply pressure to the opposing muscle groups to see whether my body needed this supplement or rejected it. It may sound bizarre, but it really worked for me. Kinesiology is noninvasive and more accurate than any other method I have used to help me assess what my body needed at that time. Using this method, we determined that I needed a digestive aid with pancreatic enzymes. We were also able to determine what vitamins I needed and which brand of vitamin A, C, or E, I could take. All of these started to help me detoxify my body.

The biochemistry of the body is constantly changing, and as we heal our chemistry shifts. What works now may not work down the road. So it is good to have an ongoing relationship with an alternative practitioner. I stayed with mine for two years going weekly. But eventually I decided to learn how to do the kinesiology so that I could test myself at home. I continued to see my chiropractor, but less often until I saw him only once a month. Now I go to him only when I need him. When I first learned about kinesiology, he told me that I would not be able to do it on myself because it would not be objective enough. But I told him that a person must believe in something and I believed that I could get the correct answers. With practice I became more and more accurate. With this tool, I was able to gain back control, to take back the power to heal myself that I had given away.

After improving my diet and digestion, I evaluated my elimination patterns. Although it may seem normal for some people to eliminate every other day or every third day, it is unhealthy. If a person does not eliminate at least once a day, foods begin to ferment inside, thus putting more toxins into their system—toxins the body must struggle to eliminate. I took a series of colonics, approximately eight over a two-month period, to detoxify my bowels. I still take a colonic once or twice a year. I also take herbs occasionally to keep the bowels regular.

With all of the following—a clean environment, a clean diet, proper digestion, and daily elimination—my body began to detoxify itself. What is detoxification? Essentially, the body rids itself of toxins through the liver, the kidneys, the lungs, the colon, and the skin. If these organs are not working up to par, the body is unable to get the toxins out of the system. As a result, these toxins can spill over into the blood, nervous system, respiratory system, and lympathetic system, stressing the entire body.

When my body started detoxifying, it seemed as if my symptoms were worsening. But it was really my body going through a *healing crisis*, which eventually passed. If the crisis became too severe, I would cut back my detoxifying supplements and exercise less to allow my body to come back into a more even balance.

From the time I started detoxifying until I got well was about two years. Detoxification is not an overnight cure, but it does teach patience and perseverance—patience to give the body time to heal itself once it begins to detoxify and perseverance to pursue various modalities until you find one that works best for you.

During my annual pap smear, the doctor, who knew I had begun doing alternative therapies, discovered to his surprise that the adhesions that bound my rectum to my left ovary had completely disappeared. He was amazed that adhesions, which I had for 14 years, were gone. He said that if he ever got sick he would come see me, and we both laughed.

At one point, I looked into the possibility of being allergic to my own hormones. It seemed as if I became more symptomatic just prior to my periods. I found a clinical ecologist in Dallas, who tested me for the different hormones—estrogen, progesterone, luteinizing hormone, and testosterone—to see how my body responded to each one. I do not remember to which one I was allergic, but I had to take a serum sublingually underneath the tongue. The problem was that the serum seemed to worsen the symptoms, so I elected to let the hormones slide at this time. I did, however, continue eating organic meats which the clinical ecologist had recommended. He explained that when we ingest a substance with hormones, such as regular meat we buy in the supermarket, it interferes with our own hormone functioning. After switching to organic meats, I noticed I was much less symptomatic during my periods.

Along with cleaning up my environment and my diet, I began to clean up my thoughts. This was a major breakthrough. I had detoxified my body and the *condition* was gone, but could I keep it away?

I learned how to meditate and to keep my physical body aligned with a higher power than myself. For me, the higher power was God, but it does not have to be a religious figure. Through meditation, I began clearing parts of my consciousness. As a result, I was able to gradually take control of my life again. I was more at peace with my Self. I was able to get more in touch with my mind/body connection, and a whole new world was opened up to me.

I used specific positive statements, such as "I want the scar tissue surrounding my fallopian tubes to be healed." I also visualized the scar tissue shrinking and asked for new and healthy cells and tissue to take its place. One of the oldest books in the world says—ASK and Ye shall receive.

It has been two years since the doctor told me that he no longer detected any endometrial adhesions. I am healthier than I have ever felt before. But my goal for this year is to be even healthier still. Once you lift the barriers that keep you trapped in your own mindset, the sky is limitless!

Illness: A Call to Change

Jo Blanche Dutcher *46*
Milford, Pennsylvania
Diagnosed with endometriosis in 1984

I have had menstrual pain all my life. But in June 1984, at age 38, I started to have a different kind of pain. Six doctors and six months later, I had a diagnostic laparoscopy that revealed moderate endometriosis. Within those six months, the pain had grown considerably and extended from my lower back down the backs of my thighs for at least two weeks each month, from ovulation to onset of menses. Standing for any length of time, for example at a cocktail party or while visiting a museum, quickly became unbearable.

As I write this, it has been almost eight years since the diagnosis. At that time, videolaser laparoscopy was in its infancy. I had never heard of it and it was unavailable in New York City. So my laparoscopy was outpatient surgery for diagnosis only, not removal of endometriosis. Afterwards, my doctor recommended that I take Danocrine (danazol) for nine months. In looking back, I am amazed at how the treatment options have grown in a relatively short period of time. More importantly, I am amazed at how much *I* have grown in terms of my management of the disease on the psychological, physical, emotional, and even spiritual levels.

1985

I went on danazol for nine months, from January to September. Overall, I did well on it. My dosage was 200 mg, four times daily. In anticipation of possible weight gain, I watched my diet, joined a health club and exercised regularly. Danazol's steroidal effect actually put me in great shape!

The lack of pain and premenstrual syndrome made me more energetic and I felt good. I did have some hot flashes, but on the recommendation of a friend I used a prescription topical liquid product called Drysoldobomatic, which within several weeks of regular use eliminated the problem completely. For the vaginal dryness, I used Lubrin, an over-the-counter suppository. I also experienced occasional acne in the form of large cysts for which I visited a dermatologist. The most troublesome side effect was a bladder infection that I got in June. Despite one antibiotic after another, it would not clear up. By late August the only option left was hospital-strength antibiotics. At that point I stopped taking the danazol and the infection slowly cleared, although it did take many more months for the bladder sensitivity to disappear.

When my period resumed, I had no pain. It was wonderful! The vaginal dryness disappeared. Unfortunately so did the exceptionally firm muscle tone, though I continued to work out regularly.

Psychologically that first year and a half was difficult. I had faced challenges in my life before, but there had been nothing to prepare me for the overwhelming loss of control that I felt when I learned that I might have an incurable illness. In fact, for several years I referred to endometriosis as a *condition*, not an illness. As the pain intensified and spread, I became fearful for my quality of life. In retrospect, I think that at some deep level I may have thought there must be something wrong with me as a person to have gotten this disease. I rarely had let that thought penetrate my conscious mind, but I do think it was lurking around in my psyche somewhere.

I knew there was no known cure for endometriosis and often felt despair at the thought of living in pain for the next 10 to 15 years until menopause. Suddenly the fact that my mother and her sister had gone through menopause relatively late in life no longer seemed advantageous. Just as people were once afraid to tell others that they had been diagnosed with cancer, I told very few people about my endometriosis. I felt that in my male-dominated workplace, any mention of my having *female problems* would hinder my career progress. Making the rounds of doctors trying to get an accurate diagnosis and treatment plan was physically and emotionally exhausting. I stressed myself further by trying not to let any of this interfere with my job responsibilities.

My parents and brother were sympathetic, but their experience was with illnesses for which one could take medicine and get better. They seemed to have no grasp of the despair unleashed by the chronic nature of the disease. While intellectually they knew I was in pain, their expectations of me, in terms of how much I could do physically and how balanced and even-tempered I ought to be emotionally, did not change. And my expectations of myself did not change much either.

The local chapter of the Endometriosis Association was a wonderful source of support. It was through the Association that I first heard of a renowned Atlanta-based physician's pioneering work with videolaser laparoscopy. In 1985 women from the New York chapter started going to Atlanta for surgery. Each time, we would gather in someone's apartment several weeks later to view the videotape. Actually *seeing* the disease, the adhesions, the damage caused to various organs, and the precision of the laser was invaluable.

In meeting these other women, I was also struck by how normal we all looked, despite the pain and other problems we were enduring. I realized that there was no outward evidence of the disease to constantly remind our friends and families of how poorly we might be feeling.

1986

Although I remained pain-free into 1986, as time went on I became increasingly exhausted at the time of my period. I was traveling a lot on business and felt subfunctional for half of each month. So in April I flew to Atlanta to have a videolaser laparoscopy. The doctor found Stage IV endometriosis and thick adhesions tying my left ovary to both my bowel and my rear pelvic wall. I took Danocrine (danazol) for two months preoperatively and three months postoperatively. Although the dosage was the same as the year before, this time I struggled with frequent breakthrough bleeding and was advised to increase the amount to 1,200 mg daily. At that level I felt sluggish and depressed.

After the surgery I returned quickly to work and resumed traveling. I can see now that I gave myself virtually no time to heal and struggled with a deep underlying exhaustion for months. Nonetheless, this period was pivotal for me. Seeing the extent of the disease in my body, even after what had appeared to be nine successful months of drug therapy, was the catalyst that led me to decide that, to some extent, I would have to become my own doctor.

I began researching theories related to the possible cause of endometriosis. During the summer, I ordered and read all the back issues of the Endometriosis Association's newsletter. The ones dealing with the yeast connection struck a chord. In addition, I read the two "bibles" on the topic—*The Missing Diagnosis* by Dr. Orian Truss and *The Yeast Connection* by Dr. William Crook. I took the self-assessment questionnaire in the front of the latter book and scored very high, which reinforced my own sense that this was an area worth investigating.

In October I had my first appointment with a doctor whose name was mentioned in one of the articles I had read. I felt fortunate to be exploring this avenue at a time when, as a result of the surgery, I could be confident that I was relatively disease-free. Dr. B explained that while in his experience there seemed to be a definite link between candida overgrowth and endometriosis, exactly what that link was is still unclear. My objective was to see whether the anti-yeast regimen could help my body to at least retard, if not entirely prevent, a recurrence of endometriosis. The regimen consisted of three components: a yeast-free diet, antifungal medication, and steps to restore a depleted immune system.

The prescribed diet was similar to that of Dr. Crook. I have found that each doctor and book suggest a slightly different diet. Such subtle differences can be confusing. I believe the important thing is to decide with your doctor what diet is best in your specific case and then stick to it. Because so many women told me that dairy products seemed to contribute to female reproductive problems, I also eliminated them from my diet, although that was not a requirement of the anti-candida program.

The diet took discipline and commitment. I followed it strictly for three years, and it caused a lot of subtle changes in my life. I cooked for myself more often, including daily lunches for work and even my own food for airplane trips. I learned to eat in advance of a party or other occasions where I might not be able to find food compatible with my diet. My family and the man I was dating at the time were very supportive in trying to accommodate my dietary requirements. My gynecologist did not give credence to the yeast connection, but neither did he discourage me from doing whatever I found helpful in managing the disease.

In addition to the diet, I took the antifungal drug, nystatin, gradually working up to one-half teaspoon of powder taken in water four times daily. In terms of medicaton, I stayed on nystatin for more than one year. Then I took Nizoral, which was very effective, for two months. For the next eight months, I took fungizone, which I obtained from France.*

The third area of treatment involved restoring my immune system. I was tested for vitamin, mineral, and essential fatty acid deficiencies via several blood and urine analyses. I was surprised at how deficient I was in some of these nutrients, such as zinc and

* Fungizone is known as oral amphotericin B in the United States and is now available is a drug called Diflucan, which has the strength of Nizoral but fewer side effects.

magnesium, which are common deficiencies in
individuals with candida. Ironically, during the same
time period I had a biannual corporate physical and
was declared exceptionally healthy! I was placed on
the following supplements: a form of B6 called
pyridoxal 5 phosphate, B1, zinc piccolinate, evening
primrose oil, Omega 3 fish oil, prescription-strength
folic acid, prescription-strength magnesium, a thyroid
extract, and an anti-oxidant supplement. As these
deficiencies began to be corrected, I really felt a
difference in my well-being.

Over the next two years, Dr. B and I explored most
of the areas mentioned in *The Yeast Connection*.
Thyroid, amino acid, and essential fatty acid
imbalances were all gradually corrected. In addition, I
was tested for allergies to mold, dust mites, grains, and
candida using skin tests, and for food allergies using
blood tests. For a time I gave myself weekly
desensitization shots for molds, dust mites, and
candida.

These various tests and interventions were not done
all at once, but gradually over two years. I learned
how important it is in medical *detective work* to
initiate only one or two changes at a time. Only in that
way was I able to notice the effect on my body and to
isolate what was helping or hindering. This type of
approach involves the doctor and patient working
together as true partners. Because it is gradual, it
requires patience and the willingness to make a
long-term change. I saw the first benefits within several
months. I had much more energy and the sensitivity in
my bladder *finally* disappeared. Usually a prime
candidate for the flu every winter, I sailed through the
winter of 1987 (and most since then) without
succumbing. The spaciness and fatigue I used to
experience with my menstrual period also disappeared.

1987

Since the 1986 surgery, I had been troubled by pain in the lower left sacral area. My doctors reminded me that although the surgery had been via laser, it still had been major surgery and that as my internal organs healed, the pain would probably diminish. It did not.

Early in 1987 I went to San Francisco on an extended business trip. Several friends there recommended that I try acupuncture. The progress that I was making on the anti-candida program probably gave me the courage to try other, complementary therapies. Once I would have been afraid, but now I figured, "Why not?"

I had acupuncture treatments at least twice a week at the outpatient clinic of the American College for Traditional Chinese Medicine in San Francisco. The Chinese doctor who treated me explained that in China acupuncture is almost always given in conjunction with herbs. He said that Western doctors who learn acupuncture rarely are willing to invest the time necessary to learn the complexities of the Chinese herbal formulas and actions. As a result, in the United States, acupuncture is frequently given without herbal medicine.

The needles themselves barely scratched the surface of my skin. I felt nothing at the insertion site. But the pain in my left sacral area intensified during the treatment even though there were no needles placed in that region. They might be placed in my knee or foot, but I felt the pain in my lower left back. I realized that there had to be some truth to what I had heard about energy, known as "chi" in Chinese, being transported along meridian pathways in the body.

The clinic had an herbal pharmacy and filled my Chinese prescription with bulk herbs that I boiled on a hot plate in my hotel room to make a strong tea. I drank this twice a day. By the time I returned to New York, the pain in my back was gone. It did not recur. The same friends who had recommended acupuncture also recommended trying visualization to prevent recurrence of the disease. Although I was unaware of it, this approach was being used successfully for cancer treatment by Dr. Carl Simonton and others. Dr. Simonton, an oncologist, is the co-author of the book titled *Getting Well Again*. I really did not know what visualization was or how to do it. But by now I was open to trying new things.

While still in San Francisco, I had started to use visualization for the pain in my lower back. I had purchased several books to learn how to put myself in a relaxed state. To achieve a relaxed state, I would slow my breathing, especially the exhalation, and would focus my attention on the painful area. As I experimented, I learned that I could make the pain go away for extended periods of time. It is hard to explain exactly how I did it. I would concentrate exclusively on the pain and somehow my mind would slowly dissolve it. I did not use a specific image for my back pain.

When I began using visualization for my endometriosis, I would visualize my pelvic area free from endometriosis and adhesions. Each day I would spend time *scanning* my pelvic cavity in my mind's eye. Whenever I *saw* the beginnings of endometriosis growth or adhesions, I would remove them. The method of removal that I imaged varied over time, but I always ended the session with an image of a disease- and adhesion-free pelvis.

Despite this success in eliminating my back pain, I wondered whether I was using the visualization directed at the endometriosis correctly. So before leaving San Francisco I had a session with a licensed therapist who uses visualization with her clients. This visit gave me the confidence that I was on the right track.

Nonetheless, when I returned to New York I had a psychological adjustment. No one I knew was using these complementary therapies. Suddenly I felt isolated and lonely. While the anti-candida program was new and controversial, the fact that I was being treated by a well-respected M.D. had made it more acceptable to other people in my life. Also, I knew that some of the officers of the Endometriosis Association were having good results with a similar regimen and eventually met several women in New York who were as well.

However, my experience in San Francisco had convinced me that if I used acupuncture again, I wanted a practitioner with traditional Chinese training. The problem was I had no idea how to get a reliable referral for someone with such a background in New York. I continued the visualization and also decided that I wanted to learn how to meditate.

The challenge was to find solid, mentally healthy people with whom I could learn and talk about these techniques. I just did not know how to meet them. I was afraid that I would only encounter "kooks" and ex-hippies. Slowly and carefully I began to make connections. In the summer, I went to a one-week conference on meditation, self-hypnosis, and visualization, which gave me a solid background in a number of relaxation and visualization techniques.

1988

For most of the next year I continued with the anti-candida program and the visualization. Dr. B moved, and since he was less accessible in his new

location, I transferred to another doctor in New York
for continuing care. When Dr. B had first taken my
medical history, he had noted that my allergies had
begun almost 18 years ago after a bout of severe
dysentery during a summer of study in Spain. My new
physician had helped pioneer a new method for
checking for parasites in a sample of rectal mucous.
My test revealed giardia (a common intestinal parasite
in the United States) and an amoeba (dormant, but still
there), as well as a lot of candida. I was surprised at
the latter because I had been doing so well and I really
thought I had the yeast under control. I began taking
Paracan 144 (which is derived from grapefruit seed
extract) to eliminate the parasite. It has no side effects
and is also a strong anti-fungal. Monthly follow-up
tests showed that the parasite and amoeba were
eliminated and the amount of candida decreased to
reasonable levels.

With my new physician, I began Enzyme Potentiated
Desensitization (EPD) shots. This approach consists of
one shot every six to eight weeks for multiple
allergans, such as food, mold, and grass. It takes
between two and three years for the benefits to
manifest, so the program requires a long-term
commitment. I decided to do everything I could to
lighten the load on my immune system.

Ever since San Francisco, I remained interested in
therapies that focus on maintaining and restoring
health by bringing into balance the chi that flows
through the meridian pathways of the body and
sustains all living organisms. A friend referred me to a
professor in the graduate program at New York
University's School of Nursing and a therapeutic touch
practitioner. The practice of therapeutic touch
represents a conscious effort to draw upon the
universal life energy and direct its flow for healing.

Through her I met a practitioner of shiatsu, which is Japanese acupressure, and a chiropractor. Again, I explored only one new approach at a time, giving myself an extended period to judge the benefits of each. In the fall I began to have pain again; a dull, aching pain reminiscent of the original pain that had started me on this journey in 1984. My gynecologist told me that the endometriosis had returned. I had vowed in 1986 that I would not take Danocrine (danazol) again. After experiencing the good effects of the yeast regimen, I felt in retrospect that the drug had depressed my immune system further. I believe that is one reason why I had such difficulty resolving my bladder infection.

So I had already decided that if the endometriosis recurred, I would opt for laser surgery rather than drugs. Psychologically, it was hard to accept a recurrence and to face surgery again. However, I consoled myself with the knowledge that many other women I knew had been having surgery annually (or, in some cases, more frequently) due to rapid recurrence, despite the fact that they had stayed on continual drug therapy. In my case almost three years had passed before an apparent recurrence, and the treatment approaches I had followed were natural ones.

I managed this surgery much differently than the one in 1986. I consulted with my physician concerning what steps to take to ensure that the post-surgical antibiotics did not precipitate a new overgrowth of candida. In addition, I ordered a two-tape audio cassette set, *Successful Surgery and Recovery*, narrated and produced by Dr. Emmett Miller, a renowned educator and lecturer specializing in stress management and psycho/physiological medicine. One tape is used daily before surgery, the other after surgery. Together they promote relaxation and a positive attitude as well as development of healing imagery specific to one's own surgery. In this way, they encourage the mind to support the body in healing and recovery.

I returned to Atlanta for the surgery in order to have continuity of care by one surgeon, who graciously agreed to my bringing a small cassette player into the operating room. I went under anesthesia listening to my favorite music and awoke to it in the recovery room. Someone on the surgical team had kindly placed it on my pillow near my ear and turned it on.

When I awoke, my brother told me that there had been no recurrence of endometriosis and relatively few adhesions. My left ovary was attached to my lateral pelvic wall by adhesions. Apparently an existing fibroid tumor had enlarged somewhat and when my uterus swelled each month, it pressed against my bladder.

I was euphoric. I felt that this news was an affirmation of all that I had done. Since I had not authorized a myomectomy and the fibroid was in a difficult position, it was left intact. The adhesions and two small cysts were vaporized with the laser.

Because of scheduling constraints, I remained in Atlanta two full days after the surgery before returning to New York. The extra day of rest was helpful. The day after arriving home, I had a masseuse come to my apartment and give me a Swedish massage. It eased and relaxed my body after all it had been through. Several days later I had a shiatsu session, also at home. And I listened to Dr. Miller's tape repeatedly. Finally, this time I told my employer that I was having minor surgery and I did not rush back to work. All of these strategies greatly assisted my healing and speeded my recovery.

The fact that the endometriosis had not recurred was an overwhelming affirmation for me. I realized that the fear of what could have been developing within my body was a major influence on my perception of the pain and the danger. The ache, now properly diagnosed, was tolerable, and I began to use visualization to shrink the fibroid, as I once had for the endometriosis.

1989–1993

In the winter of 1989, a Yale University doctor lectured to the local Endometriosis Association chapter about Lupron (leuprolide) and the use of magnetic resonance imaging (MRI) to diagnose endometriosis. She showed us slides of the MRI scans, and I was astonished at their clarity. I realized that if I had had an MRI the previous fall, I probably could have avoided surgery. It would have ruled out a large endometrioma and shown the position and growth of the fibroid. I decided to continue my endometriosis management using holistic therapies, with the addition of an MRI scan, if needed, to clarify what was happening internally.

During the past three years I have continued with these therapies. The essence of my program has not changed, but aspects of the complementary therapies continue to evolve. My father died in 1990, and as I went through a time of grieving I found that I could no longer adhere so rigidly to the anti-yeast diet. While I still follow it quite closely, I will occasionally have something made with yeast or sugar. My shiatsu practitioner moved out of state, but I found a wonderful acupuncturist, a registered nurse who graduated from a four-year program in Traditional Chinese Medicine. Acupuncture and therapeutic touch,

along with occasional chiropractic adjustments, are
currently my primary holistic therapies. I believe
consistency is crucial. For a while I did both regularly.
Now I alternate and find I am able to assess for myself
when I am *out of balance* energetically.

The long-term commitment to the EPD shots has
paid off. I have experienced a great reduction in my
seasonal allergies. The fibroid has not grown any
further. In fact, an MRI scan I had undergone in April
1992 showed that the tissues in the center of the
fibroid were actually dying. To date, I have had four
MRIs. Small cysts or endometriomas that appear on
one MRI are gone in the next. The MRIs have taught
me that in some instances my body had the strength to
take care of problems on its own. I shifted my job
responsibilities and ended a relationship. Those steps
were not easy, but I realized that in order to heal I had
to make some important changes in how my life was
structured. Some of those changes are still in progress.

In 1992, I learned another significant lesson about
how illness conditions our attitude and judgment. For
about six months, I had increasing pain in the left
sacral area. It was different from the pain I had had
after the 1986 surgery. I felt that there was a strong
chance that the endometriosis had returned or that my
left ovary was again adhered to the pelvic wall.
Chiropractic provided partial relief. But it was almost
as if the pain had two components: one structural and
one internal or *organic*. An MRI showed no evidence
of endometriosis. On the one hand, that was a relief,
but I decided that there *must* be undetected small
implants causing the pain. To my delight, I had begun
to skip menstrual periods, and blood tests confirmed
that I was definitely peri-menopausal. But I knew that
I could not live with the degree of pain for another
year or two. Reluctantly I began to prepare myself for

another surgery. It was depressing. I fell into the trap
of being hard on myself for somehow having *failed*.

My gynecologist recommended that I see an
orthopedist to rule out the possibility of any back
problems before having surgery. I was dubious. The
x-rays were all negative, but the orthopedist suggested
that since I had sprained my back two years earlier, a
lot of my difficulty might be residual weakness. He
offered a choice of the drug Naprosyn or physical
therapy. Despite my doubts, I opted for physical
therapy to strengthen my back, figuring it could not
hurt. Those sessions made all the difference. It turned
out that indeed most of the pain was structural, and as
the therapy progressed, the pain disappeared.

Now when my estrogen cycles high, which
sometimes results in spotting, I experience a throbbing
in my left sacral area. It is the *organic* kind of pain,
albeit mild and occasional. I think that it may be
endometriosis. But it is a minor, occasional pain, now
that the larger, structural component has been
alleviated. How conditioned we become to believe that
all our pain and most of our problems are
endometriosis!

God and nature have smiled on me by bringing me
menopause earlier than my mother and aunt. Thus far
it has been easy, virtually no annoying symptoms but
lots of extra energy that used to be sapped by my
periods. My interest in imagery has grown. After two
years of part-time graduate study at New York
University in New York and Duquesne University in
Pittsburgh, I have become certified in Guided Imagery
and Music Therapy. Currently, I am completing the
requirements for biofeedback certification. Recently I
also began to study herbal medicine and have learned
to make infusions, ointments, and tinctures. This work

with plants and the outdoors has brought me much pleasure.

I now understand the nature of health and healing far better than I did when I was first diagnosed. We need to be willing to incorporate the best that each medical and healing tradition has to offer. Without the twentieth-century miracle of the laser, my story would not be the same. Personally, I doubt that any complementary therapy or allopathic drug alone could have eradicated the Stage IV disease that I had in 1986. But I also doubt that laser surgery alone would have kept me disease-free for so long. There is much that centuries-old wisdom from other cultures can teach us about the true nature of health and health maintenance. And there are Western pioneers in the study of the immune system and the power of the mind that have a lot to contribute to conventional scientific medicine.

Dr. Sidney Baker wrote in his book, *Notes on the Yeast Problem, Essays and a Yeast Free Diet*, that "Illness is a signal to change. In the midst of discomfort and uncertainty some individuals are able to make changes in their direction, or in their interests or occupation, or in their relationship with themselves or with other people or in their spiritual awareness and then overcome illness to which others succumb. Change requires courage and information."

I believe that *everything* we do to help ourselves helps our health.

Endometriosis, Holistic Medicine, and Me

Marcie Katler *33*
Tempe, Arizona
Diagnosed with endometriosis in 1985

Like thousands of other women, I have been living with endometriosis for many years. Although I had been experiencing gynecological problems for a few years, it was not until my gynecologist performed a laparoscopy in May 1985 that Stage II endometriosis was confirmed. The gynecologist cauterized most of the implants, but because I had endometriosis in the cul-de-sac and because I wanted to preserve my fertility (I was only 24), he prescribed Danocrine (danazol) for six months.

That same year, I began seeing a medical doctor, John, who is also a licensed homeopath. (The state of Arizona is one of the few states that licenses homeopathic physicians.) I was seeing John for chronic illnesses other than the endometriosis. These included myofascial pain syndrome, migraines, and allergies.

The side effects from the Danocrine were so horrendous that, even though I absolutely detest needles, I agreed to let John try acupuncture to alleviate the pain and discomfort caused by the drug. It worked immediately. As I left John's office, my headache had ceased. During the course of the acupuncture treatments, other side effects such as a bloated feeling, fatigue, muscle pains and mood swings abated as well. As a result I was able to continue the danazol for the full six months.

Two and a half years later, my endometriosis symptoms recurred. This time, I had a laser laparoscopy performed by a laser specialist who was referred by my gynecologist. My endometriosis had progressed to Stage IV; however, no hormones were prescribed.

While I could write extensively about my experience with endometriosis, I will instead focus on my latest brush with it and how I was able to resolve the problem by using alternative medicine. Prior to this time, I went the conventional route—drugs and surgery—to treat my endometriosis. My goal was to preserve my fertility. Although I was using alternative therapies to treat other chronic conditions, and even the side effects of danazol, I was too afraid of taking a chance to treat the endometriosis alternatively.

In October 1991, endometriosis symptoms returned for the third time. Once again, I began experiencing pelvic pain on my left side, constipation, painful bowel movements, weight gain, left lower back pain, and cramping. This went on for a few months. The symptoms were intermittent, so I was uncertain whether it was the endometriosis again or just a couple of bad cycles. Then one month a few days before my period I had intense pelvic pain all day. I really did not believe I had endometriosis again, especially since I

had just seen the gynecologist a few months earlier and
had received a clean bill of health. I made an
appointment fully expecting the gynecologist to tell me
it was just a cyst.

Unfortunately, the gynecologist suspected the return
of endometriosis and wanted to put me on Lupron
(leuprolide acetate) for six months. Because the side
effects of Lupron are similar to Danocrine (danazol), I
was far from thrilled. Although I had wanted to
preserve my fertility at all costs, I was not as willing to
so easily acquiesce to hormone treatment this time.

I was also stunned because I had sincerely thought
that I had been able to *cure* my endometriosis. (I know
the gynecologist told me that you cannot cure
endometriosis, probably because you cannot cure
something for which the medical profession does not
know the cause!) But I had been seeing John for more
than eight years now, and we had done wonders for
my overall health and well-being with alternative
therapies—acupuncture, homeopathic remedies, herbs,
Feldenkrais neuromuscular re-education and massage
therapy—and I felt healthier and happier than I ever
had. I had also done some simpler things, such as
change my diet. I greatly reduced my sweet intake,
increased the amount of fruits, vegetables, and grains I
ate, and stopped eating red meat and foods to which I
was allergic.

More importantly, because of the mind/body/spirit
work I had been doing since 1988 with John, I
believed I had come to understand the cause of my
endometriosis. I had confronted psychological issues
from childhood and acknowledged the pain and
trauma I had endured. Until this time, for the most
part, I had shut down my emotions so as not to *make*
real the trauma. While this was a viable survival
technique, I have since learned (although it took me

years to accept) that the emotions and pain did not go away because I refused to acknowledge them. Emotions, like everything else, are energy, and because I didn't deal with them straightforwardly, the energy stayed in my system, blocking my life force and causing dis-ease. With this new awareness, and John's help, I was able to deal with the trauma, and thus the blocked energy (which was a cry for help). I was able to create flowing energy and life force, ridding myself of dis-ease. Because of this new awareness, an acceptance of the mind/body connection, and the efforts I had spent to get my energy and life force flowing freely, I believed I had found my cure for endometriosis.

Upon receiving the shocking diagnosis, I made an appointment to speak with John. I asked him if we could treat the endometriosis with Traditional Chinese Medicine. In years past, I would never have suggested this. But I had learned a great deal about my body, mind, and spirit, and I was willing to try something else. I wanted to feel that I had choices and did not have to make a decision out of fear of losing my fertility. Also, I was now at a higher level of understanding and acceptance of Traditional Chinese Medicine to treat the disease. I believed in the Chinese philosophy of chi and energy meridians.

I explained to John that I did not want to ignore the symptoms because I knew they were the precursor to endometriosis. Previously, when I had endometriosis I felt dead inside my womb and pelvic area. But these days I was feeling full of light and space, and I did not want to lose that feeling. My intuition told me that I had an energy blockage in the pelvis, and my body was providing me with a physical symptom that I could not ignore, in effect forcing me to do some additional mind/body/spirit work. If I did not deal with it, then the blockage would turn into endometriosis. The greatest gift I have received from John is the belief in my instinctual abilities and my capability to communicate with my body and to know what I need. John agreed that my symptoms were an indication that I needed to do more mind/body work.

Luckily for me, John said we could do acupuncture, herbs and a specific diet. I remember asking him what was different this time from the last time the gynecologist diagnosed endometriosis. He said me. And he was right. I was not the same person, and I was much more confident in my intuition and my ability to heal myself. Still, it was nice to receive this external validation of the positive changes I had undergone. I find that I need this validation once in a while to believe the changes and progress I have made.

In Traditional Chinese Medicine, I was diagnosed as having an accumulation of cold causing blood stagnation. I received acupuncture treatments once a week to treat the energy blockage and blood stagnation. I took two herbs—Women's Rhythm and Women's Precious, in liquid form, 15 drops each three times daily—to help break up the pelvic congestion and move my energy. In addition, I refrained from eating cold foods to dissipate the accumulation of cold in my system. I also played a Hemi-Sync* tape every night to help me visualize the blockage breaking up. During this hour, I visualized the energy moving freely in my pelvis, which I saw as a beautiful garden full of

---

* Hemi-Sync is a registered trademark of The Monroe Institute in Faber, Virginia. Hemi-Sync is patterns of sound carefully blended and sequenced to facilitate the synchronization of the two hemispheres of the brain.

sunlight, open space, and green luscious grass with wildflowers. Using the tape, I talked to the symptoms and listened to what my body had to tell me. We agreed that I would do this for three months and then I would have the gynecologist re-evaluate me. If the symptoms had not ceased and the gynecologist still felt it was endometriosis, then I would have another laparoscopy. John and I decided that I would not take the Lupron regardless because it would be detrimental for the other chronic illnesses on which we were working. I was confident this was a well thought out plan that allowed me to give the alternative medicine a chance to work, yet did not ignore the situation.

Some people may think this option is too much of a hassle. It certainly does take more time and energy than a monthly shot. But I believe that if we are to truly heal then we must take responsibility for our bodies and be active partners in our healing. This energy blockage occurred because I needed to learn something from it.

Within three months, I am happy to say that the energy blockage had dissipated. When I returned to the gynecologist, he told me that I did not have endometriosis. Of course, I already knew this. He said it must have been adhesions. However, I knew that I had had an energy blockage and because I had considered myself important and took the time to listen to, and communicate with, my body, I satisfied my needs, allowing the energy blockage to dissolve. While I was ecstatic and floated out of the office, I later thought that he had wanted to put me on this drug with terrible side effects for six months. If I had listened to him, I would have endured this all for some adhesions, which the drug does not even eliminate. I am not angry with the gynecologist. In fact, I think he is a good physician and I feel fortunate to be his

patient, because many gynecologists would not have
suspected endometriosis in a 24-year-old. But he is a
conventionally trained gynecologist and can only deal
with what he knows.

My years with endometriosis and other chronic
illnesses have taught me that a world of alternatives is
available. I believe that these alternatives, for the most
part, are superior to conventional medicine. Do not get
me wrong. I do not think we should abolish
conventional medicine. It is just that I have found that
conventional medicine makes patients subservient to
their physicians and not true partners in their healing.
It does not offer the individual a chance to take control
of her own body and to heal herself.

Immune System Despair to Immune System Repair

Kristen Kaye *35*
Cary, Illinois
Diagnosed with endometriosis in 1987

I was diagnosed with Stage II endometriosis in 1987. I tried the usual routes of treatment: Danocrine (danazol), laser surgery, and Lupron (leuprolide acetate). I tolerated all the treatments pretty well, but the endometriosis always came back. In 1990 I moved from Iowa (where there was little information or understanding about endometriosis) to Chicago. That same year I began my search for answers about this mysterious, elusive, and devastating disease.

I was on a quest for all the information I could get my hands on. So I joined the Endometriosis Association's Chicago Support Group. I attended every meeting I could, as well as any kind of free lecture. I observed two things in the support group meetings that left a big impression on me and paved the way for the approach I have taken in dealing with my endometriosis. First, in all the meetings I attended I met only two women who really seemed to be in

control of their own situations. They were the only
women who did not sit at the meetings and look like
they were sick, tired, and depressed. Both of those
women had made major changes in their diets. Second,
at one meeting at which we talked about health
problems other than endometriosis, every women
except me (or so I thought at the time) had some other
kind of health problem, such as allergies, arthritis,
lupus, and Crohn's disease. It occurred to me that
these conditions could all be classified as candida
related.

My next step was to read every book I could get my
hands on about improving my health through diet, as
well as yeast and candida-related problems. I knew
immediately that I had candida-related problems and
had had them for a long time. (I had yeast infections
for years; little did I know that yeast could invade your
whole body.) So I began making changes in my diet.
The first thing I did was eliminate all sugars and
artificial sweeteners, including corn syrup, dextrose,
fructose, and Nutrasweet. That alone made a big
difference. I was much less tired and after four or five
sugar-free months my periods were much less painful.
Next, I eliminated red meat, white flour, and white rice
products. At the same time I began taking *good*
vitamins and evening primrose oil. *Good* vitamins, in
my opinion, are not the ones that you find at your
local drugstore chain or discount store. The vitamins I
took you get at a health food store. Another bonus
was that my nails became hard as rocks and started
growing really fast. They are still that way. Also, my
thirtysomething acne really improved. I began taking a
multivitamin and a multimineral. The ones I take were
recommended by the health food store owner. They
are free of sugars and common food allergens.

I read in several books that raspberry leaf tea alleviates cramps. It really works, but it has to be raspberry *leaf* tea, not just raspberry flavored tea. I drank several cups a day during my period and occasionally throughout the month. I drank it hot during cold months and iced in the summer. I bought it at the health food store, where I now spend about half of our grocery budget buying whole grains, organic vegetables, and sugar-free snacks.

Although I was certain that I had candida-related problems, I did not know how to find a doctor to treat them. In the back of some of the books I read were listings of doctors who treat candida, but I did not think I should choose a doctor from the back of a book. At the Endometriosis Association's tenth anniversary conference held in October 1990, I got a recommendation for a local environmental allergist from a presenter who spoke on candida and allergy treatments for endometriosis.

Dr. O has an office three miles from my house. I asked the chiropractor who I was seeing for chronic lower back pain if he knew of this allergist. He said that he had referred some patients to Dr. O. I called him immediately. At that time there was a three-month waiting period for new patients.

In the meantime, Dr. O sent me a 25-page questionnaire that asked questions about every part of my body, energy levels, history of symptoms, diet and lifestyle. The questionnaire also asked about personal care products that I used, such as shampoo and detergent, as well as cleaning products for the house.

The initial visit with the doctor (not waiting, testing, or talking to the nurse) lasted two and one-half hours! When have you ever had a gynecologist or reproductive endocrinologist spend even one-half hour with you? Just by talking to me, Dr. O suspected three things: thyroid problems, candida, and allergies. All three were then confirmed by blood tests. For hypothroidism he prescribed thyroid medication, which I take daily. For the candidiasis he prescribed Diflucan, which I took for three months.

Because these treatments overlapped, it is hard to say which *cured* which symptoms. But the relief of the symptoms was immediate. Specifically, I had much more energy. In fact, my biggest complaint about the endometriosis was that I was always tired. The reproductive endocrinologists and gynecologists who I saw all said that I just had to live with it. For the first time in my life, I could get right out of bed in the morning without hitting the snooze button three or four times. And I did not drag through the day anymore anxiously waiting for bedtime.

All my symptoms of premenstrual syndrome also disappeared. Instead of having peaks and valleys or moodiness all month long, I felt like I was on an even plane. Also, the breast tenderness, bloating, and distended belly those few days before my period disappeared.

One thing I have noticed, though, is that if I cheat on my diet and eat a lot of sweets, I get a little bloated and bitchy. My husband has made all the diet changes with me, and if he eats sweets he notices he gets cranky too.

Next I was treated for allergies. Just the testing alone has taken almost three years (I was pregnant and had to postpone it for nine months). I recently completed the testing and have found out that I am sensitive to more than 80 substances, ranging from chemicals, such as formaldehyde and tobacco smoke to airborne substances, such as grass, tree pollens, and ragweed. A lot of things that I thought were symptoms of endometriosis turned out to be reactions to substances in the air or foods. For example, my lower left side used to hurt all the time. I always figured it was my left ovary. It turns out to be a reaction to wheat. As long as I eat alternative grains and stay away from wheat, I am fine. Another example are molds, which made me so tired I could hardly move. It is hard to avoid molds because they are so abundant, so I take allergy shots for the airborne allergies. It helps to avoid moldy foods, such as cheese and melons.

In addition to being treated for endometriosis for seven years, I also received numerous infertility treatments. I was given two courses of Danocrine (danazol), one in 1987 and one in 1990, and Lupron (leuprolide acetate) injections in 1989. Because I did not have a problem with ovulation, I never took fertility drugs. After seven years of traditional treatment and now two years of simultaneous alternative therapies, I decided to try in vitro fertilization. We chose zygote intrafallopian transfer (ZIFT), a procedure during which eggs were removed from my ovaries, fertilized with my husband's sperm, and returned to my tubes via a laparoscopy. During the laparoscopy, the doctor can also remove any endometriosis as long as he or she is in there. Three years earlier, I had had a laser laparoscopy and was rediagnosed with Stage IV endometriosis, with numerous adhesions and scar tissue. At the ZIFT laparoscopy, the doctor found no endometriosis and no adhesions. I truly believe it is because of the alternative treatments I used.

Now which one did it? I do not know, but I believe it was a cumulative effect. I think that each played a role, but somehow all of them together—proper diet, vitamins, evening primrose oil, and treatment for candidiasis and allergies—improved my immune system, enabling my body to keep the endometriosis away.

I also think that fat plays a role in all of this, so I am starting to work on reducing that in my diet too. I recently went back to excluding red meat entirely from my diet and also fried foods, such as chips and crackers. During the last half of my pregnancy, I began eating red meat again. I had such a craving for it I could not control myself, and the meat I usually ate—chicken—repulsed me.

The ZIFT worked on the first attempt and we now have twin girls. I recently weaned them from breastfeeding. I was lucky enough to have been without a period for almost two years now, but I was also really apprehensive about starting to menstruate again. I was more committed than ever to sticking to my healthy regimen in hopes that I would be one of the lucky ones who could keep her endometriosis from returning. After just one period, I found out that I am one of the lucky ones. I am pregnant again—this time all on my own!

Making Progress

Cindy Keck *40*
Winfield, Illinois
Diagnosed with endometriosis in 1984

From age 24 on, I had chronic back pain and I could never figure out why. I always tried to relate it to something I had done, such as lifting too much or sleeping on a soft bed. But sometimes I did very strenuous, stressful work and had no pain. Another thing that puzzled me about the ache was that heat and rest brought no relief. The pain intensified and lasted longer over the years. At times it would feel like a steel plate had covered my back side, from my shoulders to my knees.

I never associated the back pain with my menstrual cycle until at age 30 I began trying to conceive. One year later my doctor had me start charting my basal body temperature and that is when I realized the back pain peaked at ovulation.

Typically, I had heavy cramping and intestinal discomfort during my period. Often, I would have painful urination, as well. I had two or three pain-free days after my period. For the next several days, the pain was annoying, but easily masked with four to eight aspirin a day. The next ten days to two weeks I took two aspirin every four hours and was still uncomfortable. I was fortunate to be working only part-time and could make it through my normal working hours. I always felt extremely tired during these pain-filled days and attributed it to the stress and fatigue of coping with pain. I now realize that fatigue itself is one of my symptoms of endometriosis. I could usually work, exercise, and clean house in the morning. But by the afternoon I was tired and by the evening exhausted. I often spent my evenings lying on the couch.

Six months after being diagnosed with Stage III endometriosis by laparoscopy, I had a laparotomy. The visible lesions were excised and cauterized. Following surgery, I took Danocrine (danazol) for six months to shrink the endometrial growths and increase the chance of conception. While I was on danazol, the back pain greatly lessened. I was close to a normal activity and energy level.

Immediately after going off danazol, I took Clomid and underwent artificial insemination with my husband's sperm for several cycles. When no pregnancy resulted, we decided to stop pursuing infertility treatments after more than three years of trying. I had reached my limit of emotional stress. We had applied for adoption and within a year we adopted a baby girl. Two years later we adopted a baby boy.

During these years, the back pain and fatigue symptoms gradually returned until I was taking 14 or more aspirin a day for nearly ten days of each cycle. I asked my gynecologist for stronger medication for the back pain, but he recommended a hysterectomy and double oophorectomy to eliminate the endometriosis entirely. "We'll put you on hormones the day of the surgery," he said. "You'll never even know you had a hysterectomy." I decided that at 35 years of age I did not want to make that choice. I did not go back to him again.

So I began searching for alternative methods to cope with the back pain, which I now knew was attributed to my endometriosis. I read in the book *Overcoming Endometriosis* by Mary Lou Ballweg, president of the Endometriosis Association, and in association newsletters about various alternative treatments some women found successful. With young children at home, I was especially interested in something that did not involve regular trips to a practitioner's office. Taking evening primrose oil (EPO) to stop the production of prostaglandins seemed the most economical alternative in terms of both money and time. I found EPO available in most health food stores, at a cost of $35 to $40 for a bottle of 250 capsules. The recommended dosage is three to six capsules daily, but I began taking two a day because they are still relatively expensive.

At the same time I began taking Vita-Lea, a daily food supplement produced by the Shakeley company. It is essentially a comprehensive multivitamin, but it is called a "food supplement" because it is extracted from food sources and not built from chemical compounds. I take two tablets a day, but it is also available in liquid form. I also take alfalfa tablets because alfalfa is supposed to strengthen a person's immune system. It contains trace amounts of naturally occurring nutrients for which there is no U.S. recommended daily allowances. These include vitamin K, boron, chromium, manganese, and molybdenum. I take five to seven of these tablets a day. Adding the cost of the

EPO and the food supplements, I spend about $40 a
month.

During the first year, I did not notice any real
improvement, but that did not surprise me. I assumed
it would take a long time for my body to get stronger
and move toward healing. By the end of the first year,
the number of days of intense pain lessened. This trend
gradually continued.

Now, after five years of the routine, I sometimes
notice a tightening of my back muscles near the time of
ovulation. But sometimes there is no discomfort at all.
I now have up to five days a month when I take two
ibuprofen in the morning, but usually do not have
enough discomfort to take a second dose later in the
day. I no longer have painful urination during my
periods. I still have heavy cramping and frequent
diarrhea at the beginning of my period, so I do not
claim that the endometriosis is cured. I am still
annoyed by low energy levels, but have decided to
cope with that by avoiding stress as much as possible
and learning to accept a quieter lifestyle. I continue to
take the food supplement, alfalfa, and EPO daily, as I
do not want to risk returning to my previous state of
pain. I continue to grow stronger and more energetic
as time goes on.

I believe these products have given me a safe,
natural means of controlling the majority of my
endometriosis symptoms. I will continue to take them
as long as I can afford them.

Return to Balance: A Journey to Healing from Endometriosis

Lisa Kurth *35*
Alpharetta, Georgia
Diagnosed with endometriosis in 1988

For me, endometriosis is an illness that represents imbalance. To understand how I came to this conclusion, I must share what my life was like prior to my diagnosis.

Two years before I became syptomatic, my husband and I had relocated to southern California from a small, Colorado ski town. The move was big and scary, but we agreed that we needed something more to offer our daughter who was now two years old. She was so full of life, bright, inquisitive, and beautiful. Like most children, she provided joy to us when life was difficult.

While living in Colorado, I had worked as a therapist with adolescents and had begun to pursue some post-graduate studies in psychology. But after having my daughter, I chose to stay home with her instead of returning to work. Our days were spent with other young mothers and their children. We

discussed carrot salads and laundry detergents. I was
bored to tears.

One day I told my husband that I could not
continue this lifestyle. Life was not challenging enough
for me. I was pulling my hair out of my head (actually,
the stress was making it fall out in gobs). I loved our
child and had always dreamed of being the perfect
mother. I wanted to be a mother who stayed home,
baked cookies, sewed frilly dresses, made natural baby
food, and so on. But the reality of that dream was far
different and there was something missing for me. My
gut said it was time for something more. I wanted to
go back to school. I needed to learn and be in an
environment that surpassed purely domestic duties.

Thankfully my husband understood and was
supportive of me. I applied for a master's degree in
psychology at a university which was conveniently
located within walking distance from our
two-bedroom apartment. I was accepted almost
immediately. With a clinical background in child and
adolescent psychology, I was given credit for my years
of experience in the field, and I headed up the class in
clinical expertise. Fellow students consulted me on
their supervised cases. I was respected, challenged,
growing and I loved it!

Meanwhile, money was getting tight. My husband
was a freelance art director, and there were periodic
financial windfalls and lulls. Too often it seemed, the
lulls had the heavier hand. School (not to mention
child care) was expensive. So I accepted a position in a
residential treatment center for emotionally disturbed
adolescent offenders.

I provided counseling for groups, individuals,
couples and families in this state-of-the-art treatment
setting that utilized a multidisciplinary approach to
treating adolescent offenders. The program combined

mental health professionals, correctional officers, and educators in a unique team approach within a singular setting. It was an exciting opportunity to participate in a history-making program that had never been done before. I dealt with multicultural gang members and was exposed daily to every foul word imaginable. I tolerated the typical juvenile criticisms of being "too old, ugly and fat-legged." I was verbally and physically threatened, sometimes dodging objects thrown as weapons, and much more. In spite of the risks, I loved what I was doing. I was once again challenged. I was working in a field that I knew well, and I was making a difference. This was my element.

So here I was, juggling my marriage, a tight budget, a two-year-old, a job in a *jail*, and what was fast becoming a strenuous graduate degree program. I began to feel anxious. My heart raced and I worried there was not enough time for everything that had to get done. On weekends I was absorbed with school, writing papers or doing research. When I was not studying for tests, I was planning my next paper. My daughter whined constantly because I was unable to spend as much time with her as she wanted. My heart ached when I left for work in the mornings. I felt challenged, yet guilty and confused. I felt like I was missing out on being a mom and on life itself. I decided to double up on classes so I could finish the master's program faster. "If I speed up this process," I thought, "I will have more time with my family."

I was cramming a three-year program into two years. Life became so hectic I remember thinking, "My middle name should be Hurry." My husband noticed how quickly I was moving through school and urged me to slow down. I would respond all the more determined, "I'm going to finish this degree if it kills me!" Little did I know, my body was listening. . . .

When I first became symptomatic, I thought I was just having bad gas. Then I decided it must be back trouble. The pain was oddly inconsistent and seemed to radiate up my rib cage. I mentally diagnosed myself daily, wondering if I had some rare form of cancer or a hyperactive tapeworm. Then the pain would go away, sometimes as abruptly as it would appear. I wondered if I was imagining it all . . . was this happening because of STRESS?

The pain first appeared in twinges and seemed to happen unpredictably. After several months, I began to notice it worsened the week before my period was due. Right before I would bleed, the pain would feel like the back labor I experienced in giving birth to my daughter. I had been diagnosed with ovarian cysts before, so I wrote it off the pain as a *functional cyst* that would resolve itself, and continued my stressful schedule. But the back pain grew worse and changed locations. The pain began to change sides as if my uterus was a teeter-totter. I felt tired and bloated. At times the pain was so intense that it hurt to walk. Lying down gave me some relief. I took over-the-counter pain medications, which gave me minimal relief, but I found it hard to fall asleep because of the pain. After a night of restless sleep, the pain would reappear in full glory. I began treating myself with hot baths and showers. I even used a hot water bottle and a heating pad. Despite my efforts at nursing myself, the pain persisted. Worried, I decided to see a doctor.

We had not been in California long enough to secure specialists so I guessed at where to start and wound up at the office of our family physician who had recommended earlier that I discontinue using birth control pills since we were trying to have a second child. It was shortly after I stopped the Pill that these symptoms had begun (although I did not make this connection until months later). This doctor treated my now monthly *bladder infections* and *occasional cysts* with a variety of antibiotics for nearly four months. Because this treatment brought little or no relief, he referred me to a gynecologist who immediately performed a laparoscopy on me to drain a large cyst. Two weeks later, on New Year's Eve, I wound up in an emergency room because the pain was so intense. My gynecologoist insisted there was no reason for this type of pain and suggested that I see another doctor.

Over the next year, I searched frantically for an explanation of my pain, meeting with a variety of specialists, including an orthopedist, a gastroenterologist, a kidney specialist, a chiropractor, a urologist, and many others. After one year, eleven doctors, a wide range of tests, and an assortment of medications, I was finally accurately diagnosed by a university gynecologist who recognized the endometriosis that had apparently been missed in the first surgery.

When I first heard I had endometriosis, I was not completely sure what it meant, but it sounded like a confusing and big enough term to fit what I had been so intensely suffering from. At last I had an explanation for this strange, unwelcomed process that had happened in my body. Now that I had a name for it, I could begin to cope.

My journey to healing began with the sudden realization that my lifestyle needed to change. The surgery itself had required that I slow down and take care of myself. I needed to focus on *me*. I began to educate myself about endometriosis and illness in general. I read every book, brochure, and medical journal I could get my hands on. I desperately wanted to understand and gain a sense of control of what had happened to my reproductive system, to my body. Through my reading, I quickly learned that most illnesses, including endometriosis, occur as a result of faulty immune system functioning related to life stress and poor coping skills. I had simply done too much, too fast, and my immune system had talked back. Endometriosis was my body's way of saying "Stop!"

I began looking at how much work I was DOING and how little time I had just BEING. School and work had consumed my life. I had not allowed for much play or rest with my family, or even simple, self-nurturing time alone. Metaphorically, I saw my life as a scale heavily tipped to one side. I was imbalanced.

As a therapist, I was great at teaching other people to cope with life's difficulties, but I had disregarded my own needs for too long. I needed to learn how to pace myself and go slower. School and work were important, but not at the risk of harming my body.

Feeling too threatened to stop all of my activities at once, I began cutting back slowly. I scheduled time on the weekends to spend with my family, a few hours at first, and later, whole days. I also took more time to nurture myself, especially in the evenings, after work and school. I found that simple pleasures like reading something non-academic, going for a swim, or soaking in a hot jacuzzi brought me peace of mind and relaxed my muscles.

It was difficult at first to make lifestyle changes. Changing my behavior required changing my thinking. I realized how much of a perfectionist, critical thinker I had been, expecting myself to be a super student, super mom, super everything! It was not physically possible. The changes I had to make really began with giving myself permission to slow down and perform tasks with less-than-perfect results. I saw that it was my own standards I was trying to meet and no one else's. I was the person hardest to please. Simple tasks like allowing myself to buy my daughter's birthday cake from a bakery versus making it from scratch were difficult for me. But I learned to breathe deeply and recognize the joy in her face when she saw her cake. I had provided it, and that was all that mattered. She did not care where it came from.

Beginning there, I started to be more assertive, setting limits and delegating duties to others who could help. I allowed this to occur. It meant things might not meet my standards of excellence, so I had to re-evaluate those as well. I saw that while I was expecting perfection in myself, I was also expecting it in others around me. This made for strained relationships and frequent disappintments on my part. This perfectionistic attitude definitely had to go!

I began to focus more on nurturing myself. I concluded that by doing this, I would feel less stressed, happier, and thereby positively enhance my immune system functioning.

In addition to cutting back on activities, I stopped eating the sweets (chocolates in particular), fast foods, and carbonated drinks I had been consuming in such large quantities. I replaced the latter with herbal teas of all flavors, and increased the amount of fruits, vegetables, fish, and chicken I ate. I also began to drink more water to flush out my body, thinking, "I will wash it on the inside as I do on the outside."

I began taking a range of vitamins and minerals including beta carotene, a B-complex vitamin, vitamin E, calcium, magnesium, zinc, and iron. I took evening primrose oil and dong quai, too. I was careful to consume these in reasonable doses so as to maintain balance in my system.

I started a regular exercise program of sorts. I walked or moved for 20 minutes a day, at least three

times a week. I found that staying active made me feel
more rested, and I slept better at night.

I also began using imaging techniques in which I
pictured myself and my reproductive system as
healing. This process, similar to that being successfully
used with cancer patients, includes using deep
breathing and relaxation, along with guided imagery.
Twice a day, I would visualize my organs as healthy,
vibrant, feminine, and free from dis-ease. In my
imagery, I frequently invited my immune system to join
in the process of strengthening and maintaining health
within my body. I imagined cells as "soldiers who
guard the fort," correcting and redirecting any
confused blood flow. Now when I experience my
period, instead of dreading or fearing it, I go with the
flow. I imagine menses as a natural release of all that is
old and unnecessary, making way for new, vibrant,
healthy tissue. I include affirmations with this imagery,
using positive self-statements like "I am strong,
healthy, and balanced."

I also discovered that by better organizing and
managing my time, I could schedule short, relaxing
breaks throughout the day and get tasks completed
more effectively. For example, instead of studying in
my apartment, I took my books to a hot tub and
soaked up sun while I mastered statistics. Then I
rewarded myself with a self-nurturing activity, like
reading poetry or listening to mellow music. Quite
simply, I stopped overdoing and racing. By conserving
my energy, I was resting better, sleeping better, and
feeling happier.

During this process of self-healing, it became clear to
me that my job needed to change, as well. I felt
overstressed by this type of work, and it did not seem
to support my goal of taking care of myself. So I took
a great risk, left my job and set up a private practice.

My focus of work wandered away from gang work and delinquency and unfolded into health psychology (I now specialize in women's gynecological health issues). I wanted other women to know what I had learned about myself, my body, stress and its relationship to this difficult, challenging illness.

This process of self-healing did not happen overnight. It was a gradual metamorphosis for me. It took a great deal of education, soul searching, faith, hope, trust, patience, and a willingness to take risks and change. I combined this approach with good medical care provided by a physician I felt I could HEAL with. This meant becoming a RESPONSIBLE PATIENT as well. I was fortunate to find a gynecologist who respected how well I knew my own body, and who took time to listen to my concerns, answer questions and be a part of what I consider my Healing Team.

Returning to balance in my life has taken time and work, and has proven to be worthwhile. Within a couple of months after my diagnosis and beginning healthy life changes, I was feeling better. Pain was no longer a visitor. My periods seemed lighter and more regular. Because we still wanted to conceive, I chose not to go on any hormone therapy after the surgery. Instead, I focused on being in charge of my healing and began tracking my cycles. Six months after surgery I conceived naturally. About a year and a half after my diagnosis, I gave birth to our second child, a healthy baby boy.

Since that time, our family has relocated to Atlanta where my husband and I now share a private practice. Balancing this lifestyle with two young children continues to be a challenge, but now I am well equipped to cope. By staying balanced, I stay in charge of my health.

Self-healing is a process. I continue to recognize the daily need to give myself permission to make the changes necessary for my body and my immune system to stay strong and healthy. The reproductive system is a system of balance; even the organs are symmetrical. I recognize it is my duty, as the keeper of my body, to maintain this balance. When life gets stressful and I sense imbalance, I work to get myself centered and focused. I set realistic expectations and then move forward. I am challenged, yet balanced.

Native American culture considers most illnesses the result of a state of imbalance. The balance of mind and body are an intregal part of healing. What is experienced by the mind as stressful can affect the whole body. A sense of harmony is essential to maintaining a healthy immune system. It took an illness for me to see the need for greater harmony in my life. By paying more careful attention to the balance in my lifestyle, I am now healthier and stronger. Endometriosis no longer controls my life.

My Personal Health Transformation

Dee Anna P. Merz *31*
Stone Mountain, Georgia
Diagnosed with endometriosis in 1988

I first began having symptoms of endometriosis in 1986 at the age of 23. I had been to the doctor several times during that year for various ailments, ranging from mitral valve prolapse to gastrointestinal problems. In addition, I had several bouts with vaginal yeast infections.

Although my health seemed less than good, my personal life was definitely on the upswing. I had gotten engaged that September, about the time that my symptoms really began to kick in. My general practitioner repeatedly suggested that I was under stress. I explained that I was happier now than I had ever been, but she quickly reminded me how stressful getting married can be.

I was married one year later. My yeast infections and stomach problems continued, along with pelvic pain, especially during intercourse. I continued to ask my doctor if anything else could be going on, and she insisted that my problems were stress-induced. I was in her office at least once a month.

Finally, after a discussion with my aunt, I began to put the pieces together. My mother and her three sisters all suspected that they had endometriosis, and they have all had hysterectomies. Some of the symptoms my aunt described were similar to mine.

Because I lacked the telltale symptoms—heavy bleeding and cramps during menstruation—my doctor once again did not hear me. She did perform "some tests" to appease me and concluded that I had pelvic inflammatory disease. I was told that the condition was chronic and that I would just have to "live with it." At my insistence she also did a sonogram. It revealed a mass, which was later identified as a fibroid tumor. A history of fibroid tumors is also present in my family.

Shortly thereafter, I went to a local women's health resource center and began researching pelvic inflammatory disease and other gynecological disorders, including endometriosis. Through my research I discovered that the laparoscopy is the only accurate diagnostic tool for endometriosis. Finally, my doctor, who was not qualified to do a laparoscopy, referred me to a fertility specialist. The fertility specialist performed a laparoscopy in the spring of 1988 and diagnosed me with endometriosis. At that time, he removed endometrial tissue as well as several small fibroid cysts.

I was symptom-free for six months. The first symptom to recur was a stabbing pelvic pain, first detected during intercourse. For some time after sex, I had an aching, throbbing pain inside that often continued through the next day. That familiar fear shot through me and I knew what was ahead: more chronic pain and more medical examinations and procedures, which I viewed as painful, invasive, and humiliating. I continued to have pelvic pain and digestive problems throughout my cycle; I was either constipated or suffering from diarrhea. Once again, I was repeatedly diagnosed with yeast infections, even though I never had a discharge or the typical itching. Nevertheless, I was forever being prescribed that lovely tube of white gunk without ever feeling totally cured. On occasion, I would complain about the pain, which seemed to be inside my uterus, and I would be given medicine for a urinary tract infection. But inside, I knew what was going on.

In the meantime, I moved from Florida to Atlanta. Partly because of the move and partly because of financial reasons, I was not seeing one physician. I saw a nurse practitioner and then a gynecologist at Planned Parenthood. If the pain was severe, I would go to an emergency medical clinic or a family practitioner. But then I began seeing a reproductive endocrinologist I found out about through the Endometriosis Association, of which I was a member. An ultrasound revealed a cyst on my ovary. I had expressed concern about repeating surgery, so the doctor suggested that I take Danocrine (danazol) for three months. The drug removed the cyst and reduced the pain but not the stomach problems. Danocrine was expensive and had several side effects. These included weight gain, hot flashes, and severe mood swings, resulting in unexplained bouts of crying.

Within three months, the symptoms appeared again, this time with cramping and heavy bleeding. I was a full-time student working part time. I remember feeling like I just did not have time for this burden in my life. I arranged for another laparoscopy in May of 1991. I even scheduled the surgery between quarters at school. By the time I was wheeled into surgery I was begging for a hysterectomy. I had bled for 30 days straight and was not particularly impressed with my "womanhood." I just wanted my quality of life back. The surgery was completed: the doctor again removed endometrial tissue and a fibroid cyst, the latter of which had completely engulfed my uterus.

The surgery went well. My recovery was good but slow. Just days after having gone through this procedure, I was overwhelmed at the thought of having surgery again and again. I felt like I was at the mercy of the medical profession.

Shortly after my marriage in 1987, I began counseling with a therapist. Two years later, my husband and I went to marriage counseling. Although we did not have any overwhelming marital problems, we both had problems with sexual intimacy. I blamed most of my problems on endometriosis.

Within the past four years, I have come to terms with emotional, physical, and sexual abuse in my past, most of which I had repressed. When I began getting in touch with the sexual abuse, I started making the connection between my mind and body. It is no mistake that the occurrence of most of my physical symptoms coincided with the onset of my first truly intimate and committed relationship. At the time of the last surgery, I firmly believe that endometriosis was my body's way of protecting me from further abuse. Even though my husband was not a perpetrator, my body responded defensively. In my past, intimacy had equaled inappropriate sex. When I finally met someone whom I loved and respected, I did not have the proper tools to have a healthy relationship. Although the endometriosis was a physical, diagnosable, unarguable excuse, I now know the lack of sexual intimacy was a much deeper issue for both of us.

Shortly after the second surgery, I decided to try a more holistic approach to healing. I had worked on my mental and spiritual well-being, and had read much about the connection between the mind, body, and spirit. I was seeing my doctor who was treating the physical body, a therapist who was treating the mental aspects of being, and now I decided to see a chiropractor who also practices applied kinesiology to treat the body through spinal adjustments and muscle testing. Kinesiology seemed the logical balance of these three components because it stresses the health triad—believing a person should attend to the chemical, mental, and structural elements of healthful functioning. Kinesiologists use muscle testing as a diagnostic tool to treat the overall health of the body. I had gone to chiropractors for back problems, but I did not realize that they treated the entire body structurally, working with the spinal column and the nervous system to maintain function of the body.

Of course all of this is in retrospect, as I knew nothing about kinesiology and went on blind faith, having been recommended to this doctor by a respected friend. I observed and asked questions along the way, and the more I researched it the more confident I became in the path I chose. I did not feel I was at risk for bad practice because the chiropractor was highly recommended by several people who had positive results from his treatment. In fact, I figured it was either a bunch of hocus-pocus or it was something credible. I trusted my instincts, and after a year of literal new health, I did some snooping and was surprised at the schooling and credentialing of these holistic healers.

About the time I began seeing the chiropractor, in therapy I started having abreactions, which are vivid remembrances of abuse (also commonly called

flashbacks). Flashbacks can be visual, auditory, or
kinesthetic (feeling body sensations.) Mine were
kinesthetic. Soon, my visits to the chiropractor resulted
in sensational flashbacks. Often, a simple neck
adjustment would result in a writhing sensation that is
hard to put into words. The sensations were primarily
of an emotional nature. I would begin crying
uncontrollably, often my arms and hands would go
numb, and I would feel a tingly sensation throughout
my body. I would begin hyperventilating, as well. I
learned that memories are stored in the body, and
when certain parts of the body are manipulated those
memories bubble to the surface. My chiropractor was
not only aware of my physical problems, but was
attuned to my therapeutic process as well. When these
flashbacks occurred, he would gently help me through
the process and allow me to release the emotion safely,
centering me in the present before he would continue
with other chiropractic manipulations and applications
of kinesiology.

The chiropractor tested the tension of the muscles in
response to reactions to certain foods, emotions, and
supplements. For instance, the chiropractor placed a
supplement of iron under my tongue and then had me
press against his hand with my forearm. The tension
was weak, which is a sign that there is an allergic
reaction. He duplicated this forearm procedure with
food by placing food samples on my stomach as I was
lying down. When dealing with emotional stress or
trauma, he asked me to think about "the physical
abuse when I was growing up." By testing my muscle
response, he determined whether I had resolved the
conflict or whether I still had issues attached to the
trauma. Because emotions are subjective in nature, not
all kinesiologists perform muscle testing in this area. It
depends much on the philosophical slant of the

practitioner, as some chiropractors see kinesiology as
an exact science, testing only those foods and
supplements that are administered orally.
Through muscle-testing, I was diagnosed with
several food allergies. Consequently, I have removed
wheat, dairy, soy, meat and other various items, such
as vanilla, onions, garlic, caffeine, chocolate, and
coconut from my diet. My chronic digestive problems
have diminished greatly.
In addition, I was treated with various vitamins and
minerals. I was given a multi-vitamin and mineral
supplement, which I continue to take daily. I also take
bee pollen, which boosts the immune system. I have
taken vitamin B-12 supplements in chewable tablets to
aid digestion. I also have taken vitamin A and E
emulsion drops to aid in the functioning of my ovaries.
Both the B-12 and A and E drops are time-limited
supplements. The muscle-testing illuminated to the
doctor what my body needed at that particular time
for a variety of complaints, most of which centered
around my reproductive organs.
I have had several homeopathic remedies
administered as well. Although homeopathic remedies
can be administered on a one-time basis in the office,
my chiropractor recommended specific
over-the-counter remedies. For example, my
chiropractor prescribed Bach Flower remedies, which
are taken for emotional trauma. Flower remedies are
sought from the plant world to help restore vitality
and enable the person to overcome fears and worries,
which may be hindering the natural healing process.
Bach flower remedies come in a concentrated liquid
form and are administered through a dropper. I use
three or four drops under my tongue when I become
aware of stress.

I believe that my new approach to health has indeed helped my body remain symptom-free. Since I have used these methods, I have noticed many improvements, primarily with digestive problems and pelvic pain. I can remember always being tired and depressed. That too has greatly diminished. I noticed a small improvement within one month. Significant improvements were noticeable within three months. I continue to see my chiropractor once every four to six weeks, as I have from the beginning.

Nowadays, I see my reproductive endocrinologist for six-month checkups. I have not told my doctor about the alternative methods I have sought out. I do not know if this is a conscious decision on my part. I could say "Well, it has never come up." But I realize the subject would not come up unless I opened the conversation. I may have feared scorn or ridicule. I have relied heavily on myself through this process, and perhaps I did not want a negative response contaminating my faith in the healing that was taking place. Of course, expecting a negative outcome from my doctor is an assumption on my part. It is my hope that mainstream medicine and holistic forms of treatment will begin to find a common ground.

In addition to therapy and alternative healing methods, I have avidly read literature pertaining to abuse issues, spirituality, and alternative forms of healing. I have come across much of this reading material in health food stores and feminist book stores.

I cannot speak for all women; I can only speak for myself. The medical doctors are part of the journey that has led me to good health. But I believe if I had relied completely on the world of medicine without taking a look at other issues affecting my life and the options available on a holistic level, I would still be caught in the cycle of recurring endometriosis. I also believe that I have had competent guides in all aspects of my healing. My process has not been as hit-or-miss as some women have experienced. It is one thing to read about an alternative method in a book and quite another to be able to check out that method with a qualified healer.

I realize that suggesting a debilitating disease such as endometriosis could be a result of a deeper, unresolved trauma is a far stretch for some. But I do know for me, getting in touch with my inner wounds has allowed me to move past the crippling effects of endometriosis and has given me a different perspective other than that provided by the medical model. I believe a healthy combination of all the healing disciplines will better aid women in healing from this disease. I have seen many efforts in the area of emotionality and endometriosis. I am sure that eventually the research will speak for itself and many new choices will be available to women. In the meantime, I hope my personal discoveries will help those who may identify with the piece of my journey that speaks to them.

Getting Rid of the Hysteria While Keeping Your Womb

Erika Shore *25*
Brooklyn, New York
Diagnosed with endometriosis in 1992

On a Friday evening in February 1992, as I was
relaxing on the couch with a good read, I felt a
tightening pain across my lower back. When I sat up
to touch it, the sensation drew itself down through my
pelvis, as if someone was pulling a cord down and out
of me. It was not a sharp or severe pain, but it startled
me. Somehow I knew it was different from anything I
had felt before.

This moment, however brief, has served as a catalyst
in what has been a long history of health problems and
creative solutions. It was at this point that I began
what has become a strong, proactive stance with
doctors—a role that I have yet to abandon or
compromise. From the age of 13, I had been in and
out of doctors' offices complaining about irregular
periods, heavy bleeding, painful and frequent
urination, abdominal bloating, and pelvic and back
pain. Throughout the years, at one time or another, I

150

have been told that I suffer from ovarian cysts, a bladder infection, a recurrent urinary tract infection, and cystitis; that I don't ovulate; and even that I have an overactive imagination and deep psychological problems—my mother should beware. Countless doctor visits, unpleasant tests always coming up negative, and medications that failed to bring relief, all propensity to think for myself and to ask a lot of questions.

It was in this state of mind that I considered the unusual pain in my back, and what I should do about it. My symptoms rapidly became acute and I found myself unable to do the things I had always enjoyed doing, such as taking long walks in the city, lifting weights, and going to museums and films. It took four months for me to agree to a laparoscopy, which led to a diagnosis of endometriosis.

The first thing my doctor suggested as a course of medication was the Pill, taken continuously. This, she said, would produce a pseudo-pregnancy state and force my symptoms into remission. While I had taken the Pill for contraceptive purposes in the past, I had always responded poorly to it, falling prey to a host of menacing side effects. But because it was relatively harmless and less expensive than the other available medications, I decided to try it. Also, it was familiar to me, and this provided an enormous comfort. I remained on the Pill, switching prescriptions and physicians twice over the course of six months. During this time, I bled almost constantly, experienced debilitating back and pelvic pain, and began passing blood clots when I urinated. I also lacked energy. As if these symptoms were not enough, I was angry and resentful that I had gained 15 pounds, despite almost constant nausea. (I found that red raspberry leaf tea, available in health food stores, worked remarkably well for nausea. I would drink at least two cups a day, especially during meals.) A sufferer of migraines since the age of 14, I had terrible headaches while I was on the Pill, not to mention skin problems and irrational mood swings. I quickly became depressed, daunted by the reality of a chronic disease that I could not understand.

The one thing I did during this time that changed the course of my treatment more than anything else was read. I read all the books and articles about endometriosis I could find. I joined a support group and attended lectures. I talked to everyone I could about it, learning from their knowledge and experience. Through this self-education I gained strength and confidence, and I learned to trust myself and make my own decisions. It was only then that I could embark on the road to health.

Through my research, I found that the over-whelming response to controlling the disease was a two-pronged approach: drug therapies and surgery. These strategies were largely directed toward the problem of infertility, and not pain relief. While I was concerned and even frightened by the prospect of infertility, I had thought long and hard about how I wanted to live my life and what I wanted to get out of it. At 24, childbearing was not an ambition of mine. It was not even something I thought about on a daily basis. Now doctors were haranguing me to consider my options and make my choices carefully. They spoke as though my chances for childbearing were rapidly passing me by—unless I tried to get pregnant in the immediate future, I might not be able to do it at all. Suddenly I found myself thinking about an issue that was deeply personal, and yet, still foreign to me. I kept asking myself what I would do if, against all odds, I got pregnant right then. Would I want to have a baby and raise a child, dramatically changing the course of my adult life? In an effort to come to terms with my desires and ambitions, I decided that even if this hypothetical pregnancy was my only shot at having children, I wasn't ready or willing to go through with it. The question of fertility, I decided, would have to wait until I was ready to consider pregnancy a real option, even if it took me ten years to reach that point.

Given my distrust of the mainstream medical establishment, it is not surprising that I was intrigued by so-called alternative treatments. During a visit to the West Coast, I learned that an aquaintance of mine had also been recently diagnosed with endometriosis. She had been in Vancouver, Canada, where she paid a visit to an herbalist, hoping to find an alternative to the conventional drug therapies. My friend gave me the business card of the herbalist, who is a member of the National Institute of Medical Herbalists. I hesitated, still drawn by the authority of conventional medicine. Breaking away from established methods is difficult, even though I did not fully believe in them. Finally, I decided to contact her.

During our initial telephone conversation, Chanchal requested that I send her a detailed summary of my health problems, including an explanation of my endometriosis symptoms, a medical history, a three-day description of my diet, and what she called a "top-to-toe review." The latter was basically a general summary of how I am feeling *everywhere*, from head to toe. I wrote a ten-page report, which we discussed during our second phone conversation. Chanchal was concerned with all aspects of my health and lifestyle, not just the gynecological issues for which I had contacted her. She asked about my job, what it required of me physically and how happy I was with it. She also wanted to know about sources of stress in my life, both physical and emotional. I felt the exchange of ideas was both thorough and mutual.

Feeling confident of her ability to help me, I began herbal treatments in early December, just a few weeks after going off the Pill. Although Chanchal did not urge me to go off the Pill, I had decided it was causing me more harm than good and so decided to stop taking it.

The herbal formula I take is basically designed to regulate my periods and heavy bleeding, as well as alleviate the pelvic and back pain. She has used herbs that act as ovarian balancers, uterine tonics, pituitary balancers, painkillers, and general relaxants. These have included camomile to relieve stress and to aid with digestion, false unicorn root and pasque flower to normalize ovarian function, yarrow to act as a decongestant and astringent, and jamaican dogwood to relieve pain. Chanchal makes the herbal formula, which consists of a tea that I drink two to three times daily. Every four to six weeks as the formula runs out, we communicate by phone to discuss my health. We talk about how I have been feeling, if my period was heavy or light, if it came early or if I had spotting in between. She also asks how my diet has been, how active I have been, and whether I have resolved a specific conflict at work. Based on our discussion, she may adjust the formula.

When I first began the treatments, Chanchal explained that it would take four to six weeks before I noticed a change. She warned that at first I might not be able to describe the improvements specifically, but that I would feel different. What she predicted came true! By mid-January I felt a shift in how I was feeling. The most notable changes were how I carried myself, my energy levels and my abdominal pain. I had become accustomed to chronic pelvic and back pain—

I had felt pain every day, doing every activity, even
sitting and walking. After six weeks on the herbs, the
pain had eased slightly. I did not feel as debilitated,
and every day I found myself able to do a little bit
more. If I was walking, I could go farther without
tiring. If I was standing, I could go a bit longer
without resting. Generally, whatever the activity, my
endurance was a bit higher.

O ver time, my periods began to come regularly
every four weeks, for the first time in more than ten
years. This did not happen with the first cycle. It took
nearly seven months. Sometimes my periods are still
heavy, and at times, painful, but even this is an
improvement over my earlier condition. Instead of
feeling pain every day, now I have it only with my
period. Rather than bleeding three weeks out of every
month, now I bleed for five to seven days, once a
month. Chanchal and I continue to address these
changes and other issues in my treatment, but thus far
the results have been enormous.

While I can boast about the effects of the herbs, and
I would not change my course with them for anything,
these results did not come from the herbs alone.
Chanchal also advises me on my diet and nutrition, as
well as vitamin and mineral supplements. On her
recommendation, I have altered my diet for an
anti-yeast regimen, also known as an anti-candida diet.
Chanchal explained that yeast is a simple organism
which lives in the body naturally, most notably in the
digestive tract and the vagina. Candida is a specific
type of yeast that exists in our bodies in balance with a
host of other organisms. If this balance is
upset—which can occur for several reasons including a
poor diet and exposure to antibiotics—the candida can
proliferate, bringing on chronic symptoms that often
resemble those produced by endometriosis. In my case,

these included pelvic pain, abdominal bloating, urinary symptoms (both frequency and urgency in urination), headaches, recurrent vaginal yeast infections, low energy levels, fatigue, and depression.

In an effort to combat these symptoms and to clarify their root causes, I decided to try an anti-yeast diet. The first week consisted of raw foods, only vegetables, miso, plain yogurt, nuts, and seeds. During this week I also took vitamin and protein supplements, including spirulina, garlic and vitamin C, as well as acidophilus, a friendly bacteria that fights yeast and helps maintain the intestinal flora. This part of the diet serves to cleanse the body of toxins, and pave the way to recovery.

Over the next few weeks I gradually introduced cooked foods back into my diet, but avoided dairy products (except yogurt), alcohol, caffeine, sugar (including fructose), fermented foods, and any products with yeast in them. The result was an alleviation of many of the symptoms that had previously been attributed to gynecological problems. Most notably, my abdominal bloating and low energy levels significantly improved. Over time, I have been able to add back small amounts of certain foods. Now I eat two to three pieces of fruit a day, dairy products once or twice a week, and small amounts of unrefined carbohydrates and protein. In addition, I try to eat a variety of fresh and cooked vegetables and drink plenty of water. If I stray from these basic tenets and experience a recurrence of symptoms, I modify my diet accordingly to get relief.

Aside from the more obvious physical benefits, adhering to an anti-yeast diet has been psychologically rewarding. It is a regimen that I undertook and controlled myself, providing my own motivation and discipline. When I experienced relief, there was no question that *I* had done something to bring it about. Seeing that I held the power to heal myself, and that I could exercise that power at my will, was an invaluable lesson. Many of the traditional gynecologists had painted a bleak picture of helpless women who had no choice but to rely on an insufficient medical establishment to provide only marginal relief. More than anything, the anti-candida regimen allowed me to see that the healing process begins inside each woman and relies on her own willingness and determination to succeed.

At about the same time that I began researching so-called alternative treatments, I also began corresponding with a well-known gynecologist in Oregon who specializes in surgical treatments for endometriosis. I was intrigued by his unconventional approach for treating endometriosis, and our correspondence led to an office visit in late January. At that point, I had just begun the herbal treatments, but I was not fully convinced that they would bring about the desired results; I still believed that another surgery was inevitable.

To my surprise and great relief, the gynecologist—Dr. R—did not share this view. During the office visit, he broadened my understanding of the disease and how I might manage it. Dr. R urged me to consider a larger view of the reproductive system and hormonal function. He felt that my menstrual discomforts were not directly caused by the presence of endometriosis. A treatment program that addressed the larger issue of abnormal hormone function—rather than one like surgery that only attacks the endometrial growths—might bring greater relief of all my symptoms. He encouraged me to continue on the track that I had begun, that of alternative treatments. Admittedly, he knew little about herbal remedies, but he was supportive of my work with Chanchal. He also suggested that I try physical therapy to help alleviate the pelvic and back pain. Leaving his office I felt uplifted. Not only had Dr. R validated my own views of how I could best manage this disease, he had been thorough and forthcoming with his time and information. He shared his knowledge with me in a respectful and accessible manner, and never lapsed into the impatient and condescending tone that I had experienced so many times before at the hands of gynecologists.

Shortly thereafter, I began my search for a physical therapist. I knew that a variety of body therapies existed, but I didn't know much about any of them. My mother, who once suffered from chronic low back pain, suggested that I investigate a new massage technique known as craniosacral therapy, and gave me a book to start me on my way. After reading it, I was interested, but not convinced. I made an appointment for a consultation with my mother's physical therapist, Kathy, who had practiced this technique with much success. During the visit, Kathy took stock of my body. I told her only that I had endometriosis, with which she was familiar, and that I suffered from chronic pelvic pain. Using her hands to examine my abdomen and torso, neck and head, she told me that I had adhesions on both ovaries, the appendix and the bowel. She said that the whole area was tight and would undoubtedly benefit from some sort of body work, as she called it, to mobilize these organs and improve their function. I was astounded! She had recounted information that was almost identical to what was written on my operative report, just by examining me in a gentle, non-invasive way. The only drawback was that Kathy lives in Pennsylvania and I live in New York. However, she gave me a copy of a directory of therapists trained in the craniosacral method.

Excited by the prospect of gaining relief, and wanting to know more about how I could benefit from this technique, I contacted one of the people listed in the New York section of the directory. The first physical therapist I reached, Anjani, has a medical background that is helpful in treating gynecological disorders; massage therapists do not necessarily have training in medical fields like anatomy and physiology. Anjani incorporates not only her training in craniosacral therapy, but also her knowledge of myofascial release, shiatsu massage, oriental medicine, and visceral manipulation into our weekly sessions.

As with the herbal treatments, it took about a month before I felt a difference. At first, it was only subtle; my pelvis and abdomen felt looser, certain movements and activities were easier to perform and I found myself standing a bit taller. Then one day, about eight weeks into the treatment, I felt an enormous change. Anjani was working on my abdomen, and all in a moment, I felt my insides expanding, as if they were making extra space for something. I experienced a light and fluid sensation, the result of adhesions releasing and organs freeing themselves. In the five months since that session, Anjani has helped to release adhesions throughout my body. Following the holistic belief that one part of the anatomy is inextricably linked to all others, she manipulates my chest and neck, my back and shoulders—even my head—all the while allowing me a greater range of motion and an increased potential for endurance and strength. My physical condition naturally fluctuates, and each session addresses its own set of barriers, representing a distinct step in the treatment process.

As with my relationship with Chanchal, I feel as though Anjani and I have entered into a partnership; we share information and experiences freely and make decisions mutually. She has always respected my needs and desires, and considers all aspects of my lifestyle and well-being before beginning any session. This environment has nurtured support and trust, which has enabled me to make great strides toward what has become our common goal—a healthy and pain-free life.

Although Anjani and Chanchal have become essential to my understanding of and living with endometriosis, there are still things that I do for myself. Like the anti-candida diet, exercise is one thing that I can do entirely for and by myself. I had heard from various sources—doctors, practitioners, books, and other women with endometriosis—that exercise was like a gift from heaven; if you felt well enough to do it, you couldn't afford not to do it—so they said. My most impeding symptom had always been low back pain, which kept me from any sort of pounding, aerobic activity, as well as from lifting or carrying a substantial load. I had always liked swimming, but had never done it regularly as exercise. Several people suggested I try it; they said it would not aggravate my back pain because the water would buoy my weight, and if I was lucky, it might even alleviate some of the pain. After about six weeks of physical therapy, I decided to try swimming. It felt wonderful! I could move smoothly and unimpeded through the water, swimming for as long as my stamina would hold out, which was always longer than my pain would allow on land-based exercise. Swimming became a solace, a special treat I did for myself, entirely alone and in control. When I would get cramps or bad back pain, the first thing I would think of is to go for a swim. In less than one year, I could swim a half mile, then more.

Now I even participate regularly in other sports. I play basketball, run, go for long walks, work out at a gym, and I hope to lift weights soon. What they say about exercise is true: as soon as you feel able to do it—to do anything—you can't afford not to. It has helped me both physically and emotionally; it bolsters my self-esteem and confidence, and even raises my energy levels significantly.

In addition to my exercise routine, I have reduced my visits to Anjani to every other week. I still speak to Chanchal, and we have recently resolved to cut my dosage in half, to start weaning off the herbs. I had thought I would be on a full dosage of herbs until I was 30; now I am cutting back after only 13 months. She and I have spoken explicitly about short- and long-term goals, about life decisions, and possible changes in my lifestyle, such as going to graduate school and traveling to Africa. Naturally I need to know how my course of treatment would be affected and how flexible it could be. We agreed that I would probably always have to be on some kind of herbs, most likely a maintenance tea taken once daily. With any luck, she felt I would reach that point—of maintenance—by the end of 1993. At this time, I feel comfortable with how I am planning for the future.

With a disease such as endometriosis, you can only plan so much; there is always a certain element that lies outside your control, and I think you always have to be flexible. I have tried to prepare myself emotionally and intellectually to handle any changes that may arise. Knowing that I have the support of others, I feel as though I will be able to do just that.

As a result of my experience, I believe that alternative treatments deserve much more recognition and exposure than they currently receive. For example, I wonder why these therapies have to be called *alternatives.* It irks me that the very tools that enabled me to gain control of my disease, rather than allowing it to control me, would bear the derisive title *alternative.* I only hope that medical practitioners of all stripes rethink their preconceived ideas about how to best treat this disease that continues to debilitate millions of women around the world. Likewise, I urge those women to consider their options fully and equally when constructing a treatment program for themselves.

Reference Bibliography

The following is a list of books and articles used in researching this book.

"Acupuncture: An old debate continues." *Science News*, 134:8 (1988), 122.

Badawy, Shawky Z. A., M.D., et al. "The Concentration of 13, 14-dihydro-15-keto Prostaglandin F2a and Prostaglandin E2 in Peritoneal Fluid of Infertile Patients With and Without Endometriosis." *Fertility and Sterility*, 38: 2 (August 1982), 166–170.

Ballweg, Mary Lou. *Overcoming Endometriosis: New Help from the Endometriosis Association.* New York: Congdon & Weed, 1987.

Ballweg, Mary Lou. "Endometriosis Linked to Radiation and Environmental Pollutants in Research Studies." *Endometriosis Association Newsletter*, 13:2 (1992), 1–2.

Barasch, Douglas S. "The Mainstreaming of Alternative Medicine." *The New York Times' Good Health Magazine*, October 4, 1992: 6–10.

Beling, Stephanie, MD. "Relieving Endometriosis." *Vegetarian Times*, 180 (1992): 28–32.

Browning, James E., DC. "The Recognition of Mechanically Induced Pelvic Pain and Organic Dysfunction in the Low Back Patient." *Journal of Manipulative and Physiological Therapeutics*, 12:5 (October 1989), 369–373.

Chalem, Jack Joseph and Renate Lewin. "Managing Endometriosis Through Improved Nutrition." *Let's Live*, 57:4 (1989), 34–37.

Crook, William G., MD. *The Yeast Connection.* Jackson, Tennessee: Professional Books, 1991.

Dharmananda, Subhuti. "Treatment of Endometriosis with Chinese Miedicine," A Special Report by the Institute for Traditional Medicine Prepared for the Endometriosis Association." 1993.

Drug Facts & Comparisons. St. Louis: A Wolters Kluwer Company, 1992.

Eisenberg, David M., MD, et al. "Unconventional Medicine in the United States." *The New England Journal of Medicine*, 328:4 (January 28, 1993), 246–252.

Gorman, James. "Take A Little Deadly Nightshade And You'll Feel Better." *The New York Times Magazine*, August 30, 1992.

Grist, Liz. *A Woman's Guide to Alternative Medicine.* Chicago: Contemporary Books, 1988.

Hearn, Wayne. "Where Faith Meets Science." *American Medical News*, 36:23 (June 21, 1993), 9–10.

Helms, Joseph M., MD. "Acupuncture for the Management of Primary Dysmenorrhea." *Obstetrics and Gynecology*, 69:1 (1987), 51–56.

Inglis, Brian, and Ruth West. *The Alternative Health Guide*. New York: Alfred A. Knopf, 1983.

JoHanson, Kathleen. "Traditional Chinese Medicine and Endometriosis: An interview with Daoshing Ni, CA, DOM, PhD." *Endometriosis Association Newsletter*, 14:1 (1993), 3–7.

Kaptchuk, Ted J. *The Web That Has No Weaver*. New York: Congdon & Weed, 1983.

Langone, John. "Acupuncture: New Respect for an Ancient Remedy." *Discover*, 5:8 (1984), 70–73.

Lark, Susan M., MD. *Fibroid Tumors & Endometriosis: A Self-Help Program*. Los Altos, CA: Westchester Publishing, 1993.

Lauerman, Connie. "What Else, Doc?" *Chicago Tribune Magazine*, January 24, 1993.

Lauersen, Neils H., MD, PhD, and Constance De Swaan. *The Endometriosis Answer Book: New Hope, New Help*. New York: Rawson Associates, 1988.

Lin, He Xian, MB/BS and Susan Frosolone, CA, MSCM (Eds.). "The Treatment of Endometriosis with Traditional Chinese Medicine." *The Journal of the American College of Traditional Chinese Medicine*, 7:1-2 (1989), 31–48.

Mills, Simon, MA, and Steven J. Finando, PhD. *Alternatives in Healing*. New York: NAL Books, 1989.

Mindell, Earl. *Vitamin Bible*. New York: Warner Books, 1988.

Murray, Raymond H., MD, and Arthur J. Rubel, MD. "Physicians and Healers—Unwitting Partners in Health Care." *The New England Journal of Medicine*, 326:1 (January 2, 1992), 61–64.

Nissim, Rina. *Natural Healing in Gynecology*. New York: Pandora Press, 1986.

Olive, David L., MD, and Lisa Barrie Schwartz, MD. "Endometriosis." *The New England Journal of Medicine*, 328:24 (June 17, 1993), 1759–1769.

Orey, Cal. "Facing Up to Endometriosis: Strategies to Help Yourself." *Let's Live*, 60:2 (1992), 37–39.

Phalon, Richard. "New Support for Old Therapies." *Forbes*, 152:14 (1993), 254–255.

Physicians' Desk Reference. 47th Edition. New Jersey: Medical Economics Data, 1993.

Pincus, Jane and Wendy Sanford (Eds.). *The New Our Bodies, Ourselves*. New York: Simon & Schuster, 1984.

Rier, Sherry. "Immunological Findings in Dioxin Monkey Colony." *Endometriosis Association Newsletter*, 13:4 (1992), 1.

Rynk, Peggy. "The Healing Power of Touch." *Let's Live*, 61:4 (1993),
   58–59.
Sachs, Judith. *What Women Can Do About Chronic Endometriosis.*
   New York: Dell Publishing, 1991.
Shattuck, Arthur D., CA. "Traditional Chinese Medicine and the
   Treatment of Endometriosis." *Endometriosis Association
   Newsletter*, 14:1 (1993), 2–4.
Smith, Trevor, MD. *A Woman's Guide to Homeopathic Medicine.*
   New York: Thorsons Publishers, 1984.
Stein, Diane. *The Natural Remedy Book for Women.* Freedom, CA:
   The Crossing Press, 1992.
Ullman, Dana. "The Homeopath of the Future: Who Will It Be?" *Let's
   Live*, 61: 4 (1993), 40–43.
Ullman, Dana. "The Mainstreaming of Alternative Medicine."
   Healthcare Forum Journal, 36:6 (November/December 1993),
   24–30.
van Straten, Michael, ND, DO. *The Complete Natural-Health
   Consultant.* New York: Prentice Hall Books, 1987.
Wallis, Claudia. "Why New Age Medicine Is Catching On." *Time*, 138
   (1991).
Weinstein, Kate. *Living with Endometriosis: How to Cope with the
   Physical and Emotional Challenge.* Reading, MA: Addison-Wesley
   Publishing Company, 1987.
Westcott, Patsy, and Leyardia Black, ND. *Alternative Health Care for
   Women.* Rochester, VT: Thorsons Publishing Group, 1987.
"Will Acupuncture Relieve Menstrual Cramps?" *Patient Care*, 21:14
   (1987), 143–144.
Wood, Robert S. *Homeopathy Medicine That Works!* Pollock Pines,
   CA: Condor Books, 1990.
Xian, Cao Ling. "Endometriosis As Treated By Traditional Chinese
   Medicine." *Journal of the American College of Traditional Chinese
   Medicine*, 1 (1983): 54–57.

Selected Bibliography

The following is a list of books suggested for further reading. It is a compilation of books that the contributors to this book found valuable in their journey toward good health.

Annechild, Annette and Laura Johnson. *Yeast-Free Living.* New York: Perigree Books, 1986.

Baker, Sidney, MD. *Notes on the Yeast Problem, Essays and a Yeast Free Diet.* New Haven, CT: Gesell Institute of Human Development, 1985.

Balch, James F., MD, and Phyllis A. Balch, CNC. *A Prescription for Nutritional Healing.* New York: Avery Publishing Group, 1990.

Ballweg, Mary Lou. *Overcoming Endometriosis: New Help from the Endometriosis Association.* New York: Congdon & Weed, 1987.

Barral, Jean-Pierre and Pierre Mercier. *Visceral Manipulation.* Seattle: Eastland Press, 1988.

Bass, Ellen and Laura Davis. *The Courage to Heal.* New York: HarperCollins Publishers, 1992.

Burns, David, MD. *Feeling Good: The New Mood Therapy.* New York: New American Library, 1980.

Carlson, Richard, PhD, and Benjamin Shield (Eds.). *Healers on Healing.* Los Angeles: Jeremy P. Tarcher, 1989.

Carper, Jean. *The Food Pharmacy.* New York: Bantam Books, 1988.

Claussen, C.F., *Homotoxicology, The Core of a Probiotic and Holistic Approach to Medicine.* Baden-Baden, West Germany: Aurelia-Verlag GmbH, 1988.

Cousins, Norman. *Anatomy of an Illness.* New York: W.W. Norton, 1985.

Cousins, Norman. *Head First: The Biology of Hope.* New York: E.P. Dutton, 1989.

Crook, William G., MD. *The Yeast Connection.* Jackson, TN: Professional Books, 1991.

Crook, William G., MD, and Marjorie Hurt Jones, RN. *The Yeast Connection Cookbook.* Jackson, TN: Professional Books, 1989.

Dufty, William. *Sugar Blues.* New York: Warner Books, 1988.

Dychtwald, Ken. *Bodymind.* Los Angeles: Jeremy P. Tarcher Inc, 1986.

Ehrenreich, Barbara and Deirdre English. *Complaints and Disorders.* New York: The Feminist Press, 1973.

Ehrenreich, Barbara and Deirdre English. *Witches, Midwives and Nurses.* New York: The Feminist Press, 1973.

Estes, Clarissa Pinkola, PhD. *Women Who Run With the Wolves.* New York: Ballantine, 1992.

Gawain, Shakti. *Creative Visualization.* New York: Bantam Books, 1979.

Graham, Judy. *Evening Primrose Oil.* New York: Thorson Publishers Inc., 1984.

Grist, Liz. *A Woman's Guide to Alternative Medicine.* Chicago: Contemporary Books, 1988.

Harrison, John, MD. *Love Your Disease.* Santa Monica, CA: Hay House, 1988.

Hay, Louise. *Heal Your Body.* Santa Monica, CA: Hay House, 1988.

Hay, Louise. *You Can Heal Your Life.* Santa Monica, CA: Hay House, 1984.

Hoffman, David. *The New Holistic Herbal.* Rockport, MA: Element Books, 1990.

King, Jan. *Hormones from Hell.* Chatsworth, CA: CCC Publications, 1990.

Kroeger, Hannah. *The Seven Spiritual Causes of Ill Health.* United States: Hannah Kroeger, 1988.

Kaptchuk, Ted J. *The Web That Has No Weaver.* New York: Congdon & Weed, 1983.

Lark, Susan M., MD. *Fibroid Tumors & Endometriosis: A Self-Help Program.* Los Altos, CA: Westchester Publishing, 1993.

Lauersen, Neils H., MD, PhD, and Constance De Swaan. *The Endometriosis Answer Book: New Hope, New Help.* New York: Rawson Associates, 1988.

Levine, Barbara Hoberman. *Your Body Believes Every Word You Say.* Boulder Creek, CA: Aslan Publishing, 1991.

Macrae, Janet. *Therapeutic Touch: A Practical Guide.* New York: Alfred A. Knopf, 1988.

Maleskey, Gale and Charles B. Inlander. *Take This Book to the Gynecologist With You: A Consumer's Guide to Women's Health.* New York: Addison-Wesley & Company, 1991.

Meichenbaum, D., PhD. *Stress Inoculation Training.* New York: Pergamon Press, 1985.

Mindell, Earl. *Vitamin Bible.* New York: Warner Books, 1988.

Nissim, Rina. *Natural Healing in Gynecology.* New York: Pandora Press, 1986.

Northrup, Christiane, MD. *Honoring Our Bodies: Endometriosis.* Yarmonth, ME: Women to Women, 1990. Sound cassette.

Ordinato Antihomotoxica et Materia Medica. Baden-Baden, West Germany: Heel, 1986.

Owen, Lara. *Her Blood is Gold: Celebrating the Power of Menstruation.* San Francisco: HarperCollins Publishers, 1993.

Pitzele, Sefra Aobrin. *One More Day: Daily Meditations for People With Chronic Illness.* New York: Harper/Hazelden, 1988.

Porter, Garrett and Patricia A. Noris, PhD. *Why Me?* Walpole, NH: Stillpoint Publishing, 1985.

Reckeweg, Hans Heinrich, MD. *Homotoxicology, Illness and Healing Through Anti-Homotoxic Therapy.* Alburquerque, NM: Menaco Publishing, 1984.

Register, Cheri. *Living with Chronic Illness: Days of Patience and Passion.* New York: Bantam Books, 1989.

Rossman, Martin, MD. *Healing Yourself.* New York: Pocket Books, 1989.

Sachs, Judith. *What Women Can Do About Chronic Endometriosis.* New York: Dell Publishing, 1991.

Shealy, C. Norman, MD, PhD, and Caroline M. Myss, MA. *The Creation of Health: Merging Traditional Medicine with Intuitive Diagnosis.* Walpole, NH: Stillpoint Publishing, 1988.

Siegel, Bernie S., MD. *Love, Medicine and Miracles.* New York: Harper & Row, 1990.

Siegel, Bernie S., MD. *Peace, Love and Healing.* New York: Harper & Row, 1989.

Simonton, Carl O., Stephanie Matthews-Simonton, and James L. Creighton. *Getting Well Again.* New York: Bantam Books, 1978.

Smith, Lendon, MD. *Feed Yourself Right.* New York: Dell Publishing, 1983.

Sontag, Susan. *Illness as Metaphor.* New York: Farrar, Straus & Giroux, 1978.

Stein, Diane. *All Women Are Healers.* California: The Crossing Press, 1990.

Steinman, David. *Diet for a Poisoned Planet.* New York: Ballatine Books, 1990.

Stitt, Paul A. *Beating the Food Giants.* Manitowac, WI: The Natural Press, 1993.

Trowbridge, John Parks, MD, and Morton Walker, DPM. *The Yeast Syndrome.* New York: Bantam, 1988.

Truss, Orian, MD. *The Missing Diagnosis* Birmingham, AL: The Missing Diagnosis Inc., 1983.

Upledger, John. *Your Inner Physician and You: Craniosacral Therapy Somatoemotional Release.* Berkeley, CA: North Atlantic, 1992.

Valentine, Tom and Carole Valentine. *Applied Kinesiology.* Rochester, VT: Healing Arts Press, 1987.

Weinstein, Kate. *Living with Endometriosis: How to Cope with the Physical and Emotional Challenge.* Reading, MA. Addison-Wesley Publishing Company, 1987.

Wood, Robert S. *Homeopathy Medicine That Works!* Pollock Pines, CA: Condor Books. 1990.

Referring Organizations

The following organizations provide information and referrals to practitioners.

American Academy of
Environmental Medicine
P.O. Box 16106
Denver, CO 80216
(303) 622-9755

American Association of
Acupuncture and Oriental
Medicine
4101 Lake Boone Trail,
Suite 201
Raleigh, NC 27607
(919) 787-5181

American Association of
Naturopathic Physicians
2366 E. Lake Avenue E.,
Suite 322
Seattle, WA 98102
(206) 323-7610

American Chiropractic
Association
1701 Clarendon Boulevard
Arlington, VA 22209
(703) 276-8800

American Holistic Medical
Association/Foundation
4101 Lake Boone Trail,
#201
Raleigh, NC 27607
(919) 787-5146

American Massage Therapy
Association
820 Davis Street, Suite 100
Evanston, Illinois
60201-4444
(708) 864-0123

The Endometriosis Association
8585 N. 76th Place
Milwaukee, WI 53223
(800) 992-3636

Homeopathic Educational
Services
2124 Kittredge Street
Berkeley, CA 94704
(800) 359-9051

Institute for Traditional
Medicine
2017 SE Hawthorne
Portland, OR 97214
(800)544-7504

National Center for
Homeopathy
801 N. Fairfax Street, Suite
306
Alexandria, VA 22314
(206) 548-7790

National Commission for
Certification of
Acupuncturists
1424 16th Street N.W.,
#501
Washington, DC 20036
(202) 232-1404

Index

Grapefruit seed extract, 79
Graphites, 34
Guided imagery, 47
Gynacoheel, 70, 73, 74

H

Hahnemann, Samuel, 69
Healing crises, 94
Hemi-Sync, 118
Herbalism, 27-29, 79, 153-155
  vs. allopathic drugs, 27
  forms of remedies, 27
  and traditional Chinese
    medicine, 31-32, 61-62
Holistic practices, 110-111,
  114-120, 121-125. *See also
  specific types*
  individualized treatment, 13
Homeopathy, 33-34, 89
  case study, 67-80
  and symptoms, 72
Homotoxicology, 69
*Honoring Our
  Bodies—Endometriosis*, 76
Hormeel, 74
Hormonal system, 95. *See also*
  Estrogen levels
  balancing with traditional
    Chinese medicine, 85
Human chorionic gonadotropin,
  87
Humoral phase, 69
Hydrogen peroxide, 79
Hysterectomy, 128-129, 142

I

Ibuprofen, 73
Illness as signal for change, 113
Imagery. See Visualization
Immune system, 21, 23, 24, 73,
  91, 102-103, 121-126, 136
  related treatments, 39-41
Infertility, 31, 125, 128, 152-153
  case study, 58-66
Intestinal flora, 23

K

Katler, Marcie, 114
Kaye, Kristen, 121

Keck, Cindy, 127
Kelp, 78
Ketaconazole, 40
Kinesiology, 37, 75-76, 93, 145
Kurth, Lisa, 131

L

Lactobicillus acidophilus, 23, 55,
  83-84
Laparoscopy, 11-12, 58, 59, 82,
  97, 125, 143
  scar, 62
  videolaser, 100
Laparotomy, 68, 87
Laser laparoscopy, 12, 81
Law of Similars, 33
Leuprolide acetate, 10
Lifestyle, 131-140
Liver, 21
Lubrin, 98
Lungs, 91
Lupron, 60, 62-63, 82, 110, 116,
  119
Luteal phase defect, 85
Lymphomyocot, 75

M

Magnesium, 22, 23, 40, 78
Magnetic resonance imaging, 110,
  111
Masculine energy, 69
Masculine side effects, 10
Meadowsweet, 28
Meat, organic, 21, 65, 92, 95
Meditation, 95, 106
Melilot, 28
Menopausal side effects, 11
Menopause, 112
Menstrual cycle, 81, 127
  and traditional Chinese
    medicine, 32
Menstrual pain, 59, 81, 128
  and herbal remedies, 28
  traditional Chinese medicine,
    32
Merz, Dee Anna P., 141
Message therapy, 45-46
Milk thistle, 79
Miller, Emmett, 108
Mindell, Earl, 83

Minerals, 23, 54, 83, 137
The Missing Diagnosis, 101
Mixed chiropractic, 37
Molds, 125
Motherhood, 132. *See also*
  Pregnancy
Motherwort, 28
Motrin, 81

N

Nafarelin acetate, 10
Naprosyn, 81
Natural Living, 69
Naturopathic medicine, 52-57
Naturopathy, 34-37
*The New England Journal of
  Medicine*, 17
Nizoral, 102
Northrup, Christiane, 76
*Notes on the Yeast Problem,
  Essays and a Yeast Free Diet*,
  113
Nutrition, 21-25, 54-55, 76-78,
  84, 92, 101-103, 122,
  129-130, 137-138, 155-156
  and yeast infections, 40-41
Nux, 34
Nystatin, 40, 55

O

Office for the Study of Alternative
  Medicine, 13
Olive, 28
*Ordinato Antihomotoxica et
  Materia Medica*, 70
Organic food, 65, 92. *See also*
  Meat, organic; Nutrition
Overcoming Endometriosis, 120

P

PABA, 22
Pantothenic acid, 78
Paracan 144, 107
Pelvic inflammatory disease, 142
Pelvis organs, 39
Percodan, 81
Perfectionist attitude, 137
Pesticides, 21
Phosphorus, 34

Physical therapy, 111, 158-159
Ponstel, 81
Potassium, 22, 23
Pregnancy, 64, 85, 87, 128,
  152-153
Premenstrual syndrome, 24
Pro-gest cream, 78
Progesterone, 85, 87
Protaglandins, 21-22, 24
Psoronoheel, 74
Pulse, 32

Q

Quercetin, 55

R

Raspberry, 28
Raspberry leaf tea, 88, 123,
  150-151
Relaxation, 47, 106, 138
Rosemary, 28

S

Saunas, 79-80
Scar tissue integration therapy, 45
Selenium, 23
Self-hypnosis, 106
Sepia, 34, 73, 74
Sexual abuse, 144
Shepherd's purse, 28
Shiatsu. *See* Acupressure
Shore, Erika, 150
Short bowel syndrome, 87-88
Simonton, Carl, 105
Skin condition, 86
Spinal misalignments, 37
Sports, 161
Straight chiropractic, 37
Stress, 63, 130, 131, 133-134,
  141-142, 154
Successful Surgery and Recovery,
  108
Sugar, 122
Surgery, 11-12, 66, 82, 108-109
Sweet Chestnut, 28
Swimming, 160

About the Editor

Ruth Carol served as president of the Chicago chapter of the Endometriosis Association from 1989 to 1993. During that time, she talked to thousands of women, both from the Chicagoland area and from around the country, as well as dozens of physicians and holistic practitioners about the disease, its symptoms and treatment options. She has been writing about health care issues for seven years.

Other Women's Health Books
from Third Side Press

SomeBody to Love: A Guide to Loving the Body You Have *by Lesléa Newman.* Looking at ourselves as beautiful, powerful, and lovable— challenging what society teaches us. Empowering women to rethink our relationships with food and with people. **$10.95 1-879427-03-6**

Cancer As a Woman's Issue: Scratching the Surface *Midge Stocker, editor.* Personal stories of how cancer affects us as women, individually and collectively. **Women/Cancer/Fear/Power series, volume 1 $11.95 1-879427-02-8**

> *"If you are a woman, or if anyone you love is a woman, you should buy this book."*
> — Outlines

Confronting Cancer, Constructing Change: New Perspectives on Women and Cancer *Midge Stocker, editor.*
Women/Cancer/Fear/Power series, volume 2
$11.95 1-879427-09-5

> *"Written from an unabashedly feminist viewpoint, these essays provide much food for thought, touch the heart, and supply useful information on making decisions regarding healthcare."* — Library Journal

> *"Read it and reap."* — Chicago Tribune

To order any Third Side Press book or to receive a free catalog, write to Third Side Press, 2250 W. Farragut, Chicago, IL 60625-1802. When ordering books, please include $2 shipping for the first book and .50 for each additional book.

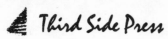 Third Side Press

The book you are holding is the product of work by an independent women's book publishing company.